Clinical and Post-Mortem Toxicology

Clinical and Post-Mortem Toxicology

Editor

Eric J. F. Franssen

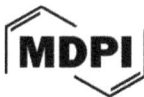 Basel • Beijing • Wuhan • Barcelona • Belgrade • Novi Sad • Cluj • Manchester

Editor
Eric J. F. Franssen
Department of Clinical Pharmacy
OLVG
Amsterdam
Netherlands

Editorial Office
MDPI
St. Alban-Anlage 66
4052 Basel, Switzerland

This is a reprint of articles from the Special Issue published online in the open access journal *Toxics* (ISSN 2305-6304) (available at: www.mdpi.com/journal/toxics/special_issues/41STYG20O5).

For citation purposes, cite each article independently as indicated on the article page online and as indicated below:

Lastname, A.A.; Lastname, B.B. Article Title. *Journal Name* **Year**, *Volume Number*, Page Range.

ISBN 978-3-7258-0694-2 (Hbk)
ISBN 978-3-7258-0693-5 (PDF)
doi.org/10.3390/books978-3-7258-0693-5

© 2024 by the authors. Articles in this book are Open Access and distributed under the Creative Commons Attribution (CC BY) license. The book as a whole is distributed by MDPI under the terms and conditions of the Creative Commons Attribution-NonCommercial-NoDerivs (CC BY-NC-ND) license.

Contents

About the Editor . . . . **vii**

Preface . . . . **ix**

Eric J. F. Franssen
Editorial "Special Issue Clinical and Post Mortem Toxicology"
Reprinted from: *Toxics* **2024**, *12*, 205, doi:10.3390/toxics12030205 . . . . **1**

Kuan-I Lee, Jing-Hua Lin, Yen-Jung Chu, Jou-Fang Deng, Wei-Lan Chu and Dong-Zong Hung
Rat Bait, Not Healthy Rice!
Reprinted from: *Toxics* **2023**, *11*, 60, doi:10.3390/toxics11010060 . . . . **7**

Elles J. Reimerink, Daan W. Huntjens, Lindsey G. Pelkmans, Jan-Willem H. J. Geerts and Eric J. F. Franssen
Successful Use of Continuous Veno-Venous Haemodialysis in a Case of Potential Lethal Caffeine Intoxication
Reprinted from: *Toxics* **2023**, *11*, 196, doi:10.3390/toxics11020196 . . . . **11**

Giuseppe Davide Albano, Stefania Zerbo, Corinne La Spina, Mauro Midiri, Daniela Guadagnino and Tommaso D'Anna et al.
Toxicological Analysis in Tissues Following Exhumation More Than Two Years after Death (948 Days): A Forensic Perspective in a Fatal Case
Reprinted from: *Toxics* **2023**, *11*, 485, doi:10.3390/toxics11060485 . . . . **17**

Lisa T. van der Heijden, Karen E. van den Hondel, Erik J. H. Olyslager, Lutea A. A. de Jong, Udo J. L. Reijnders and Eric J. F. Franssen
Internet-Purchased Sodium Azide Used in a Fatal Suicide Attempt: A Case Report and Review of the Literature
Reprinted from: *Toxics* **2023**, *11*, 608, doi:10.3390/toxics11070608 . . . . **24**

Gábor Simon, Mónika Kuzma, Mátyás Mayer, Karola Petrus and Dénes Tóth
Fatal Overdose with the Cannabinoid Receptor Agonists MDMB-4en-PINACA and 4F-ABUTINACA: A Case Report and Review of the Literature
Reprinted from: *Toxics* **2023**, *11*, 673, doi:10.3390/toxics11080673 . . . . **29**

Cristian Cobilinschi, Liliana Mirea, Cosmin-Andrei Andrei, Raluca Ungureanu, Ana-Maria Cotae and Oana Avram et al.
Biodetoxification Using Intravenous Lipid Emulsion, a Rescue Therapy in Life-Threatening Quetiapine and Venlafaxine Poisoning: A Case Report
Reprinted from: *Toxics* **2023**, *11*, 917, doi:10.3390/toxics11110917 . . . . **39**

Ivan Šoša
Quetiapine-Related Deaths: In Search of a Surrogate Endpoint
Reprinted from: *Toxics* **2024**, *12*, 37, doi:10.3390/toxics12010037 . . . . **48**

Torki A. Zughaibi, Hassan Alharbi, Adel Al-Saadi, Abdulnasser E. Alzahrani and Ahmed I. Al-Asmari
11-Nor-9-Carboxy Tetrahydrocannabinol Distribution in Fluid from the Chest Cavity in Cannabis-Related Post-Mortem Cases
Reprinted from: *Toxics* **2023**, *11*, 740, doi:10.3390/toxics11090740 . . . . **63**

Ahmed I. Al-Asmari, Hassan Alharbi, Abdulnasser E. Al-Zahrani and Torki A. Zughaibi
Heroin-Related Fatalities in Jeddah, Saudi Arabia, between 2008 and 2018
Reprinted from: *Toxics* **2023**, *11*, 248, doi:10.3390/toxics11030248 . . . . **78**

Ghassan Shaikhain, Mohammed Gaballah, Ahmad Alhazmi, Ibrahim Khardali, Ahmad Hakami and Magbool Oraiby et al.
Fatalities Involving Khat in Jazan, Saudi Arabia, 2018 to 2021
Reprinted from: *Toxics* **2023**, *11*, 506, doi:10.3390/toxics11060506 . . . . **111**

About the Editor

Eric J. F. Franssen

Eric J.F. Franssen is a hospital pharmacist and clinical pharmacologist/toxicologist. He is a registered radiopharmacist in the field of nuclear imaging and PET imaging.

Eric Franssen is the Director of Pharmacy of the Department of Clinical Pharmacy and Toxicology of OLVG Hospital (location east), a large Teaching Hospital in the centre of Amsterdam, the Netherlands. He is involved in daily patient care, including therapeutic drug monitoring, as well as clinical toxicology and post-mortem toxicology. He is the program director of the hospital pharmacy residency at OLVG Hospital (4 years of postdoctoral training program). He teaches clinical pharmacy and clinical toxicology (hospital pharmacists in residence). His research interests include clinical and forensic toxicology, therapeutic drug monitoring in critically ill patients, and radiopharmacy. He is the author of over 200 peer-reviewed articles, books, book chapters, and patents. He is a member of expert teams on clinical toxicology and post-mortem toxicology. He chairs the section Drug Analysis and Toxicology of the Dutch Foundation for Quality Assessment in Medical Laboratories. He has been the chair of the 15th International Conference of the International Association of Therapeutic Drug Monitoring and Clinical Toxicology (IATDMCT), October 2015, Rotterdam, the Netherlands. He is the chair of the clinical toxicology committee of IATDMCT (September 2021). Eric Franssen was awarded the Irving Sunshine Award for outstanding contributions in Clinical Toxicology by the IATDMCT (Rome, 19 September 2021).

Preface

Clinical toxicology and post-mortem toxicology cover a broad scientific field with many opportunities and challenges. This Special Issue addresses the opportunities and challenges of detecting the exposure and intoxications of various (recreative) drugs and novel active psychoactive drugs. Currently, an increasing number of drugs have become widely available on the internet, posing questions surrounding how and where we can detect these agents and their metabolites in body fluids, as well as what the potentials and limitations of comprehensive and targeted toxicology screenings are in clinical and forensic toxicology cases. This issue also addresses novel options for the clinical management of intoxicated patients, including the prevention of (re)absorption, the enhanced extracorporal elimination of drugs, and specific antidotes. In cases of post-mortem toxicology, how do we interpret drug levels in blood and tissues, as well as address challenges related to post-mortem redistribution and degradation?

It is our pleasure to present a Special Issue with papers covering this interesting and challenging field of toxicology.

Eric J. F. Franssen
Editor

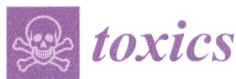

Editorial

Editorial "Special Issue Clinical and Post Mortem Toxicology"

Eric J. F. Franssen

Department of Clinical Pharmacy, OLVG Hospital, 1091 AC Amsterdam, The Netherlands; e.j.f.franssen@olvg.nl; Tel.: +31-205999111

1. Introduction

This Special Issue addresses the challenges faced in detecting the exposure and intoxications of various (recreative) drugs and novel active psychoactive drugs. An increasing number of drugs have become widely available on the internet, posing the following questions: how and where can we detect these agents and their metabolites in body fluids, and, what are the potentials and limitations of comprehensive and targeted toxicology screenings in clinical and forensic toxicology cases? This issue also addresses novel options for the clinical management of intoxicated patients: prevention of (re)absorption, extracorporal enhanced elimination of drugs, and specific antidotes. In cases of post mortem toxicology, how do we interpret drug levels in blood and tissues, as well as addressing challenges related to post mortem redistribution and degradation?

2. An Overview of Published Articles

In their case study, Lee et al. discuss bromadiolone, a potent, long-acting anticoagulant rodenticide. Bromadiolone is often blended with cereals to produce rat bait. The study outlines an incident involving six individuals employed in a small factory who suffered from a severe bleeding tendency several weeks after consuming a rice-based meal that was tainted with bromadiolone. High serum levels of bromadiolone and excessive bleeding were found in these individuals, who were then treated with vitamin K1 in the weeks following the incident. These cases indicate that long-acting anticoagulant rodenticide may induce cumulative toxicity in repeated, low-dose exposure. Blood bromadiolone levels may indicate the need for antidote therapy (Contribution 1).

Reimerink et al. describe a case of a potentially lethal caffeine intoxication after the reported ingestion of 10 g of caffeine. Due to hemodynamic instability, due to tachycardia, hypertension, and insufficient continuous labetalol infusion, the patient was started on continuous veno-venous haemodialysis (CVVHD). After successful treatment for 15 h, CVVHD was discontinued and the patient was discharged the following day. The authors stress the importance of an early recognition of caffeine intoxication, so that haemodialysis can be considered in the case of a potentially lethal intoxication (Contribution 2).

Exhumations, conducted under legal directives, are a crucial instrument in the investigation of death allegations. In cases where the cause of death is suspected to be the result of drug misuse, pharmaceutical overdose, or pesticide poisoning, this process may be applied on human remains. However, after a large postmortem interval (PMI), determining the cause of death from an exhumed body is challenging. In this issue, Albano et al. report challenges associated with postmortem drug concentration changes following exhumation more than two years after death (Contribution 3). In their case study, they present a case of a 31-year-old man who was found dead in a prison cell. During the inspection of the scene, police officers collected two blister packs—one with a tablet and the other empty. The deceased was suspected to have taken cetirizine and food supplements consisting of carnitine–creatine tablets the evening before. No relevant autopsy findings were observed. A comprehensive toxicological analysis was performed by gas chromatography coupled with mass spectrometry. The screen results were negative for substances of abuse. However, proteomic analysis returned positive results for creatine detection and negative results for other drugs (such as clarithromycin, fenofibrate, and cetirizine). The authors present the methods, and their findings, addressing the limitations of toxicological analysis in an exhumation case with a long postmortem interval (PMI).

There has been a significant increase in sodium azide intoxications since the 1980s. Sodium azide is not regularly detected in comprehensive toxicology screenings. A specific and targeted bioanalysis is required for its detection in both blood and urine. Intoxications caused by sodium azide are becoming increasingly prevalent in the Netherlands as a result of its promotion for the purpose of self-euthanasia. The mechanism of toxicity is not completely understood, but it is dose-dependent. Van der Heijden et al. present a case of suicide by sodium azide of a young woman (26 years old) with a history of depression and previous suicide attempts (Contribution 4). The deceased was found in the presence of various prescription drugs, including temazepam, domperidone—in combination with omeprazole—and the chemical preservative sodium azide. Quantitative toxicology screening of whole blood revealed the presence of 70 µg/L temazepam (toxic range > 1000 µg/L) and 28 mg/L sodium azide (fatal range: 2.6–262 mg/L). Whole blood qualitative analysis revealed the presence of temazepam, temazepam-glucuronide, olanzapine, n-desmethylolanzapine, and acetaminophen. Interestingly, in circles promoting sodium azide, it is recommended to use sodium azide in combination with medications targeting its adverse effects, such as analgesics, anti-emetics, and anti-anxiety drugs. The medicines recovered at the deceased's location, coupled with the results of the toxicology screens, appeared to be consistent with recommendations of self-euthanasia using sodium azide.

Synthetic cannabinoid receptor agonists (SCRAs) first appeared as a legal alternative to cannabis in 2004, and they have been linked to numerous fatalities since [1]. Simon et al. report a case of a 26-year-old male who died from consuming synthetic cannabinoid receptor agonists MDMB-4en-PINACA and 4F-ABUTINACA (Contribution 5). MDMB-4en-PINACA and 4F-ABUTINACA are potent synthetic cannabinoid receptor agonists (SCRAs). The scientific literature on the symptoms associated with these substances was evaluated, along with the pharmacological properties and possible mechanism of death. A forensic autopsy was performed according to Recommendation No. R (99)3 of the Council of Europe on medico-legal autopsies. Histological samples were stained with hematoxylin and eosin (HE). Complement component C9 immunohistochemistry was applied to all heart samples. Toxicological analyses were performed by supercritical fluid chromatography, coupled with tandem mass spectrometry (SFC-MS/MS) and headspace gas chromatography with a flame ionization detector (HS-GC-FID). The literature was reviewed to identify previously reported cases of MDMB-4en-PINACA and 4F-ABUTINACA use. Autopsy findings included brain edema, internal congestion, petechial bleeding, pleural ecchymoses, and blood fluidity. Toxicological analyses revealed the 7.2 ng/mL of MDMB-4en-PINACA and 9.1 ng/mL of 4F-ABUTINACA in the peripheral blood. The authors conclude that MDMB-4en-PINACA and 4F-ABUTINACA are strong, potentially lethal SCRA, and their exact effects and outcome are unpredictable.

The administration of intravenous lipid emulsion (ILE) is a proven antidote used to reverse local anesthetic-related systemic toxicity [2]. Although the capacity of ILE to generate blood tissue partitioning of lipophilic drugs has been demonstrated previously, a clear recommendation for its use as an antidote for other lipophilic drugs is still debated. Venlafaxine (an antidepressant which acts as a serotonin–norepinephrine reuptake inhibitor (SNRI)) and quetiapine (a second-generation atypical antipsychotic) are widely used in the treatment of psychotic disorders. Both are lipophilic drugs known to induce cardiotoxicity and central nervous depression. Cobilinschi at al. report a case of a 33-year-old man with a medical history of schizoaffective disorder, who was admitted to the emergency department (ED) after having been found unconscious due to a voluntary ingestion of 12 g of quetiapine and 4.5 g of venlafaxine (Contribution 6). An initial assessment revealed a cardiorespiratory stable patient, but the subject was unresponsive to a GCS of 4 (M2 E1 V1). In the ED, he was intubated, and gastric lavage was performed. Immediately after admission to the intensive care unit (ICU), his condition quickly deteriorated. He then developed cardiovascular collapse refractory to crystalloids and vasopressor infusion. Junctional bradycardia then occurred, followed by spontaneous conversion to sinus rhythm. Subsequently, frequent ventricular extrasystoles, as well as patterns of bigeminy, trigeminy, and even episodes of non-sustained ventricular tachycardia occurred. Additionally, generalized tonic–clonic seizures were observed, alongside supportive therapy, antiarrhythmic and anticonvulsant therapy, intravenous lipid emulsion bolus, and continuous infusion were administered. His condition progressively improved over the following hours, and 24 h later, he was tapered off the vasopressor. On day 2, the patient repeated the cardiovascular collapse and a second dose of ILE was administered. Over the next few days, the patient's clinical condition improved, and he was successfully weaned off ventilator and vasopressor support. The authors conclude that ILE has the potential to become a form of rescue therapy in cases of severe lipophilic drug poisoning, and should be considered a viable treatment for severe cardiovascular instability that is refractory to supportive therapy. This finding is also supported by similar papers on overdoses of venlafaxine, in which blood venlafaxine concentrations were monitored resulting in enhanced clearing of venlafaxine by ILE [3].

The pharmacokinetic features of psychoactive drugs—their significant postmortem redistribution especially—challenge traditional sampling in forensic toxicology. In response to this, Sosa performed a systematic literature review to evaluate different matrices as a surrogate endpoint in the forensic toxicology of quetiapine-related deaths (Contribution 7). This review considers the results of five comprehensive studies. The highest quetiapine concentrations were usually measured in the liver tissue. As interpreted by their authors, the results of the considered studies showed a strong correlation between some matrices, but, unfortunately, the studies presented models with poor goodness-of-fit. The distribution of quetiapine in distinct body compartments and tissues showed no statistically significant relationship with the length of the postmortem interval. Furthermore, this study did not confirm the anecdotal correlation of peripheral blood concentrations with skeletal muscle concentrations. Also, there was no consistency regarding selecting an endpoint for analysis.

An alternative matrix for post mortem toxicology analysis may be fluid obtained from the chest cavity (FCC). Zughaibi et al. studied the presence of 11-nor-Δ9-carboxy tetrahydrocannabinol (THC-COOH) in FCC of postmortem cases collected from drug-related fatalities or criminal-related deaths to evaluate its suitability for use as a complementary specimen to blood and biological specimens in cases where no bodily fluids are available or suitable for analysis (Contribution 8). The relationships between THC-COOH concentrations in the FCC samples, age, body mass index (BMI), polydrug intoxication, manner, and cause of death were investigated. Methods: Fifteen postmortem cases of FCC were analyzed using fully validated liquid chromatography-positive-electrospray ionization tandem mass spectrometry (LC-MS/MS). Results: FCC samples were collected from 15 postmortem cases; only THC-COOH tested positive, with a median concentration of 480 ng/mL (range = 80–3010 ng/mL). THC-COOH concentrations in FCC were higher than THC-COOH concentrations in all tested specimens with the exception to bile. The median ratio FCC/blood with sodium fluoride, FCC/urine, FCC/gastric content, FCC/bile, FCC/liver, FCC/kidney, FCC/brain, FCC/stomach wall, FCC/lung, and FCC/intestine tissue were 48, 2, 0.2, 6, 4, 6, 102, 11, 5 and 10-fold, respectively. Conclusion: This is the first postmortem report of THC-COOH in the FCC using cannabinoid-related analysis. The FCC samples were liquid, easy to manipulate, and extracted using the same procedure as the blood samples. The source of THC-COOH detected in FCC could be derived from the surrounding organs due to postmortem redistribution or contamination due to postmortem changes after death. THC-COOH, which is stored in adipose tissues, could be a major source of THC-COOH found in the FCC.

Urine, vitreous humor, and bile specimens are interesting alternative matrices for post mortem toxicological analyses. Al-Asmari et al. reviewed heroin-related postmortem cases reported at the Jeddah Poison Control Center in Saudi Arabia over a 10-year period (Contribution 9). Liquid chromatography electrospray ionization tandem mass spectrometry (LC/ESI-MS/MS) was utilized to determine the 6-monoacetylmorphine (6-MAM), 6-acetylcodeine (6-AC), morphine (MOR), and codeine contents in unhydrolyzed postmortem specimens. This study assessed 97 heroin-related deaths, and they represented 2% of the total postmortem cases (median age, 38; 98% male). In the blood, urine, vitreous humor, and bile samples, the median morphine concentrations were 280 ng/mL, 1400 ng/mL, 90 ng/mL, and 2200 ng/mL, respectively, 6-MAM was detected in 60%, 100%, 99%, and 59% of the samples, respectively, and 6-AC was detected in 24%, 68%, 50%, and 30% of the samples, respectively. The highest number of deaths (33% of total cases) was observed in the 21–30 age group. In addition, 61% of cases were classified as "rapid deaths", while 24% were classified as "delayed deaths". The majority (76%) of deaths were accidental; 7% were from suicide; 5% were from homicide; and 11% were undetermined. The availability of urine, vitreous humor, and bile specimens provided valuable information regarding the opioids that were administered and the survival time following heroin injection.

Interpreting potential toxicological fatalities is challenging due to lack of data on drug reference concentrations in postmortem tissues. Towards this, Shaikhain et al. investigated the autopsy findings and toxicological results of fatalities involving khat in Saudi Arabia's Jazan region from 1 January 2018 to 31 December 2021 (Contribution 10). All confirmed cathine and cathinone results in postmortem blood, urine, brain, liver, kidney, and stomach samples were recorded and analyzed. Autopsy findings and the manner and cause of death of the deceased were assessed. Saudi Arabia's Forensic Medicine Center investigated 651 fatality cases over four years. Thirty postmortem samples were positive for khat's active constituents, cathinone and cathine. The percentage of fatalities involving khat was 3% in 2018 and 2019 and increased from 4% in 2020 to 9% in 2021, when compared with all fatal cases. These cases all included males ranging in age from 23 to 45. Firearm injuries (10 cases), hangings (7 cases), road traffic accidents (2 cases), head injuries (2 cases), stab wounds (2 cases), poisoning (2 cases), unknown causes (2 cases), ischemic heart disease (1 case), brain tumors (1 case), and choking (1 case) were responsible for these deaths. In total, 57% of the postmortem samples tested positive for khat only, while 43% tested positive for khat with other drugs. Amphetamine was the drug most frequently involved. The average cathinone and cathine concentrations were 85 and 486 ng/mL in the blood, 69 and 682 ng/mL in the brain, 64 and 635 ng/mL in the liver, and 43 and 758 ng/mL in the kidneys, respectively. The 10th–90th percentiles of blood concentrations of cathinone and cathine were 18–218 ng/mL and 222–843 ng/mL, respectively. These findings show that 90% of fatalities involving khat had cathinone concentrations greater than 18 ng/mL and cathine concentrations greater than 222 ng/mL. According to the cause of death, homicide was the most common fatality involving khat alone (77%). More research is required, especially toxicological and autopsy findings, to determine the involvement of khat in crimes and fatalities. This study may help forensic scientists and toxicologists investigate fatalities involving khat.

3. Conclusions

In conclusion, this Special Issue shows the importance of comprehensive and targeted toxicology screening to detect different drugs and toxins in blood and tissues of both patients and the deceased. Quantitative measurements of drugs in body fluids are helpful in monitoring the use of antidotes and extracorporal clearance of patients in the clinic [4–8]. Additionally, reports on quantitative measurements of parent drug and metabolites in the body fluids of the deceased can enhance our knowledge of postmortal redistribution and ultimately aid in establishing a potential toxicological cause of death [9–15].

Conflicts of Interest: The author declares no conflict of interest.

List of Contributions:

1. Lee, K.-I.; Lin, J.-H.; Chu, Y.-J.; Deng, J.-F.; Chu, W.-L.; Hung, D.-Z. Rat Bait, Not Healthy Rice! *Toxics* **2023**, *11*, 60. https://doi.org/10.3390/toxics11010060.

2. Reimerink, E.J.; Huntjens, D.W.; Pelkmans, L.G.; Geerts, J.-W.H.J.; Franssen, E.J.F. Successful Use of Continuous Veno-Venous Haemodialysis in a Case of Potential Lethal Caffeine Intoxication. *Toxics* 2023, *11*, 196. https://doi.org/10.3390/toxics11020196.
3. Albano, G.D.; Zerbo, S.; La Spina, C.; Midiri, M.; Guadagnino, D.; D'Anna, T.; Buscemi, R.; Argo, A. Toxicological Analysis in Tissues Following Exhumation More Than Two Years after Death (948 Days): A Forensic Perspective in a Fatal Case. *Toxics* 2023, *11*, 485. https://doi.org/10.3390/toxics11060485.
4. van der Heijden, L.T.; van den Hondel, K.E.; Olyslager, E.J.H.; de Jong, L.A.A.; Reijnders, U.J.L.; Franssen, E.J.F. Internet-Purchased Sodium Azide Used in a Fatal Suicide Attempt: A Case Report and Review of the Literature. *Toxics* 2023, *11*, 608. https://doi.org/10.3390/toxics11070608.
5. Simon, G.; Kuzma, M.; Mayer, M.; Petrus, K.; Tóth, D. Fatal Overdose with the Cannabinoid Receptor Agonists MDMB-4en-PINACA and 4F-ABUTINACA: A Case Report and Review of the Literature. *Toxics* 2023, *11*, 673. https://doi.org/10.3390/toxics11080673.
6. Cobilinschi, C.; Mirea, L.; Andrei, C.-A.; Ungureanu, R.; Cotae, A.-M.; Avram, O.; Isac, S.; Grințescu, I.M.; Țincu, R. Biodetoxification Using Intravenous Lipid Emulsion, a Rescue Therapy in Life-Threatening Quetiapine and Venlafaxine Poisoning: A Case Report. *Toxics* 2023, *11*, 917. https://doi.org/10.3390/toxics11110917.
7. Šoša, I. Quetiapine-Related Deaths: In Search of a Surrogate Endpoint. *Toxics* 2024, *12*, 37. https://doi.org/10.3390/toxics12010037.
8. Zughaibi, T.A.; Alharbi, H.; Al-Saadi, A.; Alzahrani, A.E.; Al-Asmari, A.I. 11-Nor-9-Carboxy Tetrahydrocannabinol Distribution in Fluid from the Chest Cavity in Cannabis-Related Post-Mortem Cases. *Toxics* 2023, *11*, 740. https://doi.org/10.3390/toxics11090740.
9. Al-Asmari, A.I.; Alharbi, H.; Al-Zahrani, A.E.; Zughaibi, T.A. Heroin-Related Fatalities in Jeddah, Saudi Arabia, between 2008 and 2018. *Toxics* 2023, *11*, 248. https://doi.org/10.3390/toxics11030248.
10. Shaikhain, G.; Gaballah, M.; Alhazmi, A.; Khardali, I.; Hakami, A.; Oraiby, M.; Alharbi, S.; Tobaigi, M.; Ghalibi, M.; Fageeh, M.; et al. Fatalities Involving Khat in Jazan, Saudi Arabia, 2018 to 2021. *Toxics* 2023, *11*, 506. https://doi.org/10.3390/toxics11060506.

References

1. European Monitoring Centre for Drugs and Drug Addiction. Synthetic Cannabinoids in Europe—A Review. 2021. Available online: https://www.emcdda.europa.eu/system/files/publications/14035/Synthetic-cannabinoids-in-Europe-EMCDDA-technical-report.pdf (accessed on 24 June 2023).
2. Liu, Y.; Zhang, J.; Yu, P.; Niu, J.; Yu, S. Mechanisms and Efficacy of Intravenous Lipid Emulsion Treatment for Systemic Toxicity From Local Anesthetics. *Front. Med.* 2021, *8*, 756866. [CrossRef] [PubMed]
3. de Wit, D.; Franssen, E.; Verstoep, N. Intralipid administration in case of a severe venlafaxine overdose in a patient with previous gastric bypass surgery. *Toxicol. Rep.* 2022, *9*, 1139–1141. [CrossRef] [PubMed]
4. Moffat, A.C. *Clark's Analysis of Drugs ENS Poisons*, 3rd ed.; Moffat, A.C., Osselton, M.D., Widdop, B., Eds.; Pharmaceutical Press: London, UK, 2004; ISBN 0853694737.
5. Allen, D.; McWhinney, B. Quadrupole Time-of-Flight Mass Spectrometry: A Paradigm Shift in Toxicology Screening Applications. *Clin. Biochem. Rev.* 2019, *40*, 135–146. [CrossRef] [PubMed]
6. Maurer, H.H. Hyphenated high-resolution mass spectrometry—The "all-in-one" device in analytical toxicology? *Anal. Bioanal. Chem.* 2020, *413*, 2303–2309. [CrossRef] [PubMed]
7. Mardal, M.; Fuskevåg, O.-M.; Dalsgaard, P.W. Comprehensive UHPLC-HR-MSE screening workflow optimized for use in routine laboratory medicine: Four workflows in one analytical method. *J. Pharm. Biomed. Anal.* 2021, *196*, 113936. [CrossRef] [PubMed]
8. Caspar, A.T.; Meyer, M.R.; Maurer, H.H. Blood plasma level determination using an automated LC–MS^n screening system and electronically stored calibrations exemplified for 22 drugs and two active metabolites often requested in emergency toxicology. *Drug Test. Anal.* 2018, *11*, 102–111. [CrossRef] [PubMed]
9. Baselt, R.C. *Disposition of Toxic Drugs and Chemical in Man*, 12th ed.; Biomedical Publications: Seal Beach, CA, USA, 2020; ISBN 978-0-578-57749-4.
10. Hansen, S.L.; Dalsgaard, P.W.; Linnet, K.; Rasmussen, B.S. Comparison of Comprehensive Screening Results in Postmortem Blood and Brain Tissue by UHPLC–QTOF-MS. *J. Anal. Toxicol.* 2022, *46*, 1053–1058. [CrossRef] [PubMed]
11. Launiainen, T.; Ojanperä, I. Drug concentrations in post-mortem femoral blood compared with therapeutic concentrations in plasma. *Drug Test. Anal.* 2013, *6*, 308–316. [CrossRef] [PubMed]
12. Swanson, D.M.; Pearson, J.M.; Evans-Nguyen, T. Comparing ELISA and LC–MS-MS: A Simple, Targeted Postmortem Blood Screen. *J. Anal. Toxicol.* 2021, *46*, 797–802. [CrossRef] [PubMed]

13. Grapp, M.; Kaufmann, C.; Streit, F.; Binder, L. Systematic forensic toxicological analysis by liquid-chromatography-quadrupole-time-of-flight mass spectrometry in serum and comparison to gas chromatography-mass spectrometry. *Forensic Sci. Int.* **2018**, *287*, 63–73. [CrossRef] [PubMed]
14. Kriikku, P.; Rasanen, I.; Ojanperä, I.; Thelander, G.; Kronstrand, R.; Vikingsson, S. Femoral blood concentrations of flualprazolam in 33 postmortem cases. *Forensic Sci. Int.* **2019**, *307*, 110101. [CrossRef] [PubMed]
15. Alasmari, A.; Alhejaili, A.; Alharbi, H.; Alzahrani, M.; Zughaibi, T. Challenges and insights: Methamphetamine analysis in post-mortem putrefied human tissues in a hot climate. *Saudi Pharm. J.* **2024**, *32*, 101990. [CrossRef] [PubMed]

Disclaimer/Publisher's Note: The statements, opinions and data contained in all publications are solely those of the individual author(s) and contributor(s) and not of MDPI and/or the editor(s). MDPI and/or the editor(s) disclaim responsibility for any injury to people or property resulting from any ideas, methods, instructions or products referred to in the content.

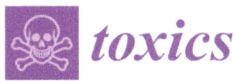

Case Report

Rat Bait, Not Healthy Rice!

Kuan-I Lee [1], Jing-Hua Lin [2], Yen-Jung Chu [3], Jou-Fang Deng [4], Wei-Lan Chu [4] and Dong-Zong Hung [2,*]

1. Department of Emergency, Buddhist Tzu Chi General Hospital, Taichung Branch, Taichung 42721, Taiwan
2. Division of Toxicology, China Medical University Hospital, Taichung 40447, Taiwan
3. Department of Emergency Medicine, China Medical University Hospital, Taichung 40447, Taiwan
4. Division of Clinical Toxicology & Occupational Medicine, Department of Medicine, Taipei Veterans General Hospital, Taipei 11217, Taiwan
* Correspondence: dzhung0224@gmail.com; Tel.: +886-4-2205-2121

Abstract: Bromadiolone, a potent, long-acting anticoagulant rodenticide is frequently tinted to a red or pink color and mixed with cereals as rat bait. Six peoples working in a small factory suffered from a severe bleeding tendency several weeks after consuming a rice meal that was tainted with bromadiolone mistaken to be healthy food. High serum levels of bromadiolone and excessive bleeding were found in these individuals, and they needed vitamin K1 therapy for weeks. These cases indicated that long-acting anticoagulant rodenticide might induce cumulative toxicity in repeated, low-dose exposure, and the blood levels of bromadiolone might be an indicator for antidote therapy if available.

Keywords: bromadiolone; rat bait; vitamin K1

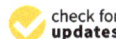

Citation: Lee, K.-I.; Lin, J.-H.; Chu, Y.-J.; Deng, J.-F.; Chu, W.-L.; Hung, D.-Z. Rat Bait, Not Healthy Rice! *Toxics* **2023**, *11*, 60. https:// doi.org/10.3390/toxics11010060

Academic Editor: Eric J. F. Franssen

Received: 7 December 2022
Revised: 3 January 2023
Accepted: 6 January 2023
Published: 8 January 2023

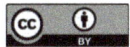

Copyright: © 2023 by the authors. Licensee MDPI, Basel, Switzerland. This article is an open access article distributed under the terms and conditions of the Creative Commons Attribution (CC BY) license (https:// creativecommons.org/licenses/by/ 4.0/).

1. Introduction

Bromadiolone, a second-generation, long-acting anticoagulant rodenticide (LAAR) with a white to yellow color chemically, is marketed worldwide and frequently colored with red dye and mixed with grains as rat bait of 0.005% *w/w* in general meaning that it might be confused with healthy food such as red yeast rice. Long-acting anticoagulant rodenticides have an extremely higher affinity to vitamin K epoxide reductase (VKOR), a key enzyme in the liver for vitamin K reactivation, compared with warfarin. The tight binding and inhibition of VKOR by LAAR allows for a significant deficiency in the reduced form of vitamin K and this is characterized by prolonged coagulopathy and bleeding after initial treatment and the need for high-dose vitamin K1 therapy after LAAR poisoning [1]. The half-life of bromadiolone in human beings has been reported to be as long as 144 h [2]. Repeated small-dose exposures had been suggested to be likely to produce cumulative toxicity and severe coagulopathy [1], but it has never been reported in the literature before. Here, we describe six individuals suffering from varied doses of bromadiolone through repeated exposure with severe bleeding diathesis due to the misuse of rat-bait rice as healthy food for weeks.

2. Case Report

Six individuals in Taiwan, working overseas from a small company in China, presented to an emergency department (ED) due to hematemesis, hematuria, and multiple ecchymoses on their skin. Tracing back their histories, the first case (patient 1) sought medical attention in a local hospital in China because of severe hematuria, gum bleeding, tarry feces, and ecchymoses for 1–2 days. An unexplained bleeding tendency with a prolonged prothrombin time (PT) was found there. His condition improved and he was released from hospital after a transfusion of fresh frozen plasma. Unfortunately, the hemorrhagic symptoms reappeared and his colleagues subsequently experienced similar symptoms. All of them went back to the emergency room under the suspicion of massive food poisoning due to LAAR-contaminated rice (Figure 1), which their cook mistook as red yeast rice and it was served three times a day. The tainted rice containing 0.5% w/w of bromadiolone was prepared to be 0.005% w/w of bait. These patients consumed 1–3 bowls of rice per meal and they had lasted for more than 2 weeks before bleeding diathesis occurred. Without rice washing, a bowl of rice is estimated to contain 9 milligrams of rat poison.

These people all denied any trauma or history of anticoagulants use. Most of them presented with hematuria, gum bleeding, and subcutaneous ecchymosis (5/6 patients). All of them were free from any signs or symptoms of central nervous system damage. Their clinical manifestations are summarized in Table 1. All of them were admitted and received intravenous vitamin K1 therapy until their INR values were normal. Twenty to thirty mg of vitamin K1 intravenously per day in divided doses was prescribed and was adjusted with the INR values being checked every 2–3 days. These patients were discharged and followed-up at an out-patient clinic while their antidotes were shifted to an oral route if they could keep their normal INR value under only 10 mg of vitamin K1 injection per day. All of them recovered with normal INR values and they were free of symptoms after vitamin K1 therapy when they were discharged from hospital. Their blood samples were taken when they were admitted and quantitated by LC-MS/MS in the Toxicology Laboratory of Taipei Veterans General Hospital [3], and high serum bromadiolone (3.9~74.5 ng/mL) levels were identified in all of these six patients.

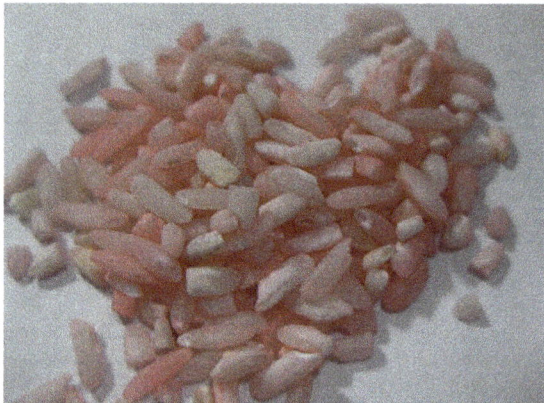

Figure 1. The appearance of the bait. The rice grains were stained unevenly by pink bromadiolone powder before being washed (the patient provided the rice grains).

Table 1. Clinical and demographic data of the six patients with bromadiolone intoxication.

	Patient 1 *	Patient 2	Patient 3	Patient 4	Patient 5	Patient 6
Age	58	32	54	32	29	27
Sex	M	M	M	M	F	M
Hematuria	+	+	+	−	+	+
Gum bleeding	+	+	−	+	+	+
GI bleeding	+	−	−	+	−	−
Ecchymosis	+	+	+	+	−	+
Conjunctival hemorrhage	−	−	+	−	−	−
PT/INR (Normal 0.8–1.2)	Unclotted	Unclotted	Unclotted	17.5/1.55	37.7/3.31	25.1/2.21
SBL	74.5	6.17	8.94	7.5	3.9 #	8.0
Total dose of Vit. K1 & (mg), IV/Oral	130/50	120/100	110/50	120/100	50/0	40/0

*: The patient consumed meals every day during that time and was lost to the follow-up after discharge. SBL: serum bromadiolone level, ng/mL, assayed by LC-MS/MS; #: The patient delayed medical attention and blood tests for three days. &: IV form 10 mg/vial and oral form 5 mg/tablet. Patient 1 was the manager for machine maintenance, patients 2 and 4 were the assistants of the manager, patient 3 was the boss, and patients 5 and 6 were the daughter of the boss and her husband, respectively. The patients 5 and 6 frequently went out on business and might have been less exposed.

3. Discussion

Bromadiolone, a kind of 4-hydroxycoumarin, is a popular LAAR [1]. Compared with the 17-h half-life of warfarin, the elimination half-life of bromadiolone in animal blood is much longer, about 1.0 to 2.4 days, and even up to 170–318 days in rat livers [1,4]. In case reports of human poisoning [2,5], bromadiolone was eliminated from the blood with the terminal half-life of 10–24 days, contrary to the first phase of 3.5–6 days. The fact of slow elimination suggests the possibility of the cumulative toxicity of bromadiolone in cases of long-term, repeated exposure, similar to the behavior of heavy metal lead or cadmium [1].

Bromadiolone is commonly prepared as a 0.5% red to pink color liquid formulation to be mixed with grains such as rice and corn to a 0.005% w/w concentration and it is commonly applied in buildings as rat bait in China [6]. Due to the colorful appearance and the lack of warning signs, it could easily be served as a meal by mistake. Rice is usually washed with water before cooking, and the concentration of leftover bromadiolone in a rice meal might be less than 0.005%. Bromadiolone is thermally stable below 200 degrees Celsius [7]. In cases without washing, a bowl of rice is calculated to contain 9 mg of rat poison. Although we did not obtain the sample for a toxin assay, it was clear from these patients' data that more serious exposure through continuous ingestion rather than intermittent exposure resulted in higher blood levels, more rapid onset, and severe manifestations. Patient 1, who consumed meals three times a day and 2–3 bowls/meal, suffered from prompt bleeding diathesis and his blood rodenticide level was found to be more than 74.5 ug/L; patient 5 with intermittent exposure and the latest presentation had the lowest blood level and required low doses of vitamin K1 therapy and subsequently had the shortest period of treatment. This suggested that long-term and repeated exposure to such small doses of bromadiolone might have also induced cumulative toxicity and led to a bleeding tendency in humans. According to these small groups of patients, the most frequent presentations were hematuria and gum bleeding with varied serum concentrations of LAAR.

Long term vitamin K1 therapy to prevent a relapse in bleeding tendency and the absence of reliable clinical indicators have been noted in acute LAAR poisoning [1,8]. A few reports from cases studies have indicated that serum bromadiolone levels less than 10 ng /mL and 4–10 ng/mL of brodifacoum are associated with a consistently normal coagulation profile without antidote therapy [1,2,5]. These findings seemed to not be applicable in these cases of low-dose and repeated LAAR exposure. The patients who suffered from significant bleeding and abnormal INR values required the use of vitamin K1 therapy even with serum bromadiolone level less than 4 ng/mL [7].

Our study has some limitations. Firstly, these patients could not correctly recall how much contaminated rice they had consumed. Secondly, we did not obtain the rice sample for a bromadiolone assay due to restrictions on the importation of agricultural products. Thirdly, we did not study the toxicokinetics of bromadiolone in these patients to define the antidotes use. However, we confirmed their bromadiolone exposure by detecting significant toxin bromadiolone levels by the LC-MS/MS in the patients' blood, and its possible relationship to exposure frequency.

In conclusion, low-dose and repeated exposure to LAARs could lead to significant coagulopathy and bleeding from the vital organs and there is a need for prompt antidote therapy regardless of the LAAR blood level.

Author Contributions: Conceptualization, K.-I.L., D.-Z.H. and J.-H.L.; methodology, W.-L.C.; investigation, D.-Z.H.; resources, D.-Z.H. and J.-F.D.; data curation, Y.-J.C., K.-I.L. and W.-L.C.; writing—original draft preparation, K.-I.L.; writing—review and editing, D.-Z.H.; visualization, J.-H.L.; supervision, J.-F.D. and D.-Z.H.; project administration, J.-H.L. and D.-Z.H.; funding acquisition, D.-Z.H. All authors have read and agreed to the published version of the manuscript.

Funding: A part of this research was founded by the China Medical University Hospital (DMR-111-218).

Institutional Review Board Statement: Ethical review and approval were waived for this study due to data included in the paper without any ID information.

Informed Consent Statement: Patient consent was waived due to NO ID information included.

Data Availability Statement: Not applicable.

Acknowledgments: The authors thank the China Medical University Hospital (DMR-111-218) for their funding. We also wish to acknowledge the emergency department staff of the China Medical University Hospital for collecting the samples.

Conflicts of Interest: The authors declare no conflict of interest. The funders had no role in the design of the study; in the collection, analysis, or interpretation of data; in the writing of the manuscript; or in the decision to publish the results.

References

1. King, N.; Tran, M.-H. Long-acting anticoagulant rodenticide (superwarfarin) poisoning: A review of its historical development, epidemiology, and clinical management. *Transfus. Med. Rev.* **2015**, *29*, 250–258. [CrossRef] [PubMed]
2. Vindenes, V.; Karinen, R.; Hasvold, I.; Bernard, J.P.; Mørland, J.G.; Christophersen, A.S. Bromadiolone poisoning: LC-MS method and pharmacokinetic data. *J. Forensic Sci.* **2008**, *53*, 993–996. [CrossRef] [PubMed]
3. Bidny, S.; Gago, K.; David, M.; Duong, T.; Albertyn, D.; Gunja, N. A validated LC-MS-MS method for simultaneous identification and quantitation of rodenticides in blood. *J. Anal. Toxicol.* **2015**, *39*, 219–224. [CrossRef] [PubMed]
4. Horak, K.E.; Fisher, P.M.; Hopkins, B. Pharmacokinetics of anticoagulant rodenticides in target and non-target organisms. In *Anticoagulant Rodenticides and Wildlife*; Springer: Cham, Switzerland, 2018; pp. 87–108.
5. Lo, V.M.; Ching, C.K.; Chan, A.Y.; Mak, T.W. Bromadiolone toxicokinetics: Diagnosis and treatment implications. *Clin. Toxicol.* **2008**, *46*, 703–710. [CrossRef] [PubMed]
6. National Center for Biotechnology Information. PubChem Compound Summary for CID 54680085, Bromadiolone. Available online: https://pubchem.ncbi.nlm.nih.gov/compound/Bromadiolone (accessed on 30 November 2022).
7. Long, J.; Peng, X.; Luo, Y.; Sun, Y.; Lin, G.; Wang, Y.; Qiu, Z. Treatment of a long-acting anticoagulant rodenticide poisoning cohort with vitamin K1 during the maintenance period. *Medicine* **2016**, *95*, e5461. [CrossRef] [PubMed]
8. Chu, Y.J.; Lin, J.H.; Hung, D.Z. Oral administration of injectable vitamin K1 in brodifacoum intoxication. *BioMedicine* **2022**, *12*, 47–49. [CrossRef] [PubMed]

Disclaimer/Publisher's Note: The statements, opinions and data contained in all publications are solely those of the individual author(s) and contributor(s) and not of MDPI and/or the editor(s). MDPI and/or the editor(s) disclaim responsibility for any injury to people or property resulting from any ideas, methods, instructions or products referred to in the content.

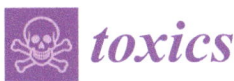

Case Report

Successful Use of Continuous Veno-Venous Haemodialysis in a Case of Potential Lethal Caffeine Intoxication

Elles J. Reimerink [1,*], Daan W. Huntjens [2], Lindsey G. Pelkmans [1], Jan-Willem H. J. Geerts [1] and Eric J. F. Franssen [2]

1 Department of Intensive Care, OLVG Hospital, 1061 AE Amsterdam, The Netherlands
2 Department of Clinical Pharmacy, OLVG Hospital, 1061 AE Amsterdam, The Netherlands
* Correspondence: elles.reimerink@gmail.com

Abstract: Here we describe the case of a potentially lethal caffeine intoxication after the reported ingestion of 10 g of caffeine. Due to hemodynamic instability with tachycardia and hypertension with an insufficient effect of continuous labetalol infusion, the patient was started on continuous veno-venous haemodialysis (CVVHD). After successful treatment for 15 h, CVVHD could be discontinued, and the patient was discharged home the next day. This case report is the first to report the use of CVVHD as a haemodialysis modality in the case of caffeine intoxication and illustrate the effect on caffeine clearance. We stress the importance of an early recognition of caffeine intoxication, so that haemodialysis can be considered in the case of a potentially lethal intoxication.

Keywords: caffeine intoxication; continuous veno-venous haemodialysis; caffeine clearance

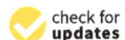

Citation: Reimerink, E.J.; Huntjens, D.W.; Pelkmans, L.G.; Geerts, J.-W.H.J.; Franssen, E.J.F. Successful Use of Continuous Veno-Venous Haemodialysis in a Case of Potential Lethal Caffeine Intoxication. *Toxics* **2023**, *11*, 196. https://doi.org/10.3390/toxics11020196

Academic Editor: Luis D. Boada

Received: 19 January 2023
Revised: 15 February 2023
Accepted: 17 February 2023
Published: 20 February 2023

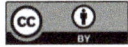

Copyright: © 2023 by the authors. Licensee MDPI, Basel, Switzerland. This article is an open access article distributed under the terms and conditions of the Creative Commons Attribution (CC BY) license (https://creativecommons.org/licenses/by/4.0/).

1. Introduction

Caffeine (1,3,7-trimethylxanthine, guaranine) is a plant-derived alkaloid that antagonizes subtype A1 and A2a of the adenosine receptor. Since adenosine is an endogenous neuromodulator with mostly inhibitory effects, the antagonism of adenosine results in positive inotropic and chronotropic effects. After oral intake, caffeine is completely absorbed in the stomach and intestines (100%) and is almost completely metabolized in the liver by CYP1A2 (95%) through demethylation of caffeine (1,3,7-trimethylxanthine) to paraxanthine (1,7-dimethylxanthine) [1]. In the case of regular consumption, the metabolization will follow linear kinetics with a half-life time of 3–5 h and a plasma protein binding of 17–36% [2]. However, due to saturation of CYP1A2 in the case of an overdose, the unbound fraction will no longer be dose-linear, and caffeine will follow non-linear kinetics, with a higher unbound fraction and a prolonged half-life time [3,4]. After metabolization, the majority of caffeine is eliminated in the urine through renal excretion (85–88%) [4].

Caffeine is usually consumed to increase focus, enhance memory, and improve physical performance [2,5,6]. Caffeinated beverages contain varying amounts of caffeine: from 60 mg in a cup of coffee to 250 mg in potent energy drinks. The consumption of these beverages rarely leads to severe caffeine intoxication. However, caffeine supplements regularly exceed this dosage and can contain 300 mg each. These supplements can be bought limitlessly online as pills or as pure caffeine powder. The increasing popularity of caffeine supplements has resulted in (unintended) severe caffeine intoxications, which have necessitated treatment in a critical care unit and even resulted in deaths [7,8]. The American Association of Poison Control Centers (AAPCC) reported 3031 cases of single-substance caffeine use in 2019, of whom 415 were treated in a healthcare facility, resulting in 23 major outcomes (life-threatening or resulting in significant residual disability or disfigurement) [9].

In previous case reports, the ingestion of 15–30 mg/kg has resulted in significant toxicity, and oral doses of >5 g have been reported as fatal [1,6]. Due to the severity of the intoxication, elimination enhancement through renal replacement therapy (RRT) can prove a valuable therapy. Since caffeine is a small hydrophilic molecule with a low plasma protein binding (17–36%) and a small volume of distribution of 0.61 L/kg, it is suitable for dialysis [10]. Successful intermittent haemodialysis has been described in case reports; however, the benefit of continuous renal replacement therapy remains unclear.

We here describe a case of severe caffeine intoxication with a potentially lethal oral dosage of 10 g, in which the patient has made a full recovery after treatment with continuous veno-venous haemodialysis (CVVHD). To the best of our knowledge, this is the first case report describing the use of CVVHD as a haemodialysis modality in caffeine intoxication.

2. Case Report

A 29-year-old male patient with a history of borderline personality disorder and alcohol and drug abuse presented to the cardiac care unit (CCU) with complaints of chest pain and stomach ache. As an experiment, he voluntarily consumed 10 g of caffeine powder approximately 14 h before presentation. About 30 min after ingestion, he started vomiting and sweating, and he experienced a heavy chest. These symptoms endured 13 h until he eventually called the emergency services and was taken to the hospital. At presentation, the patient was anxious and in pain, and he was sweating profusely. Vital signs showed tachycardia (152 beats per minute), hypertension (190/35 mmHg), tachypnoea (22 breaths per minute), an oxygen saturation of 97%, and a subfebrile temperature (38 °C). The electrocardiogram showed sinus tachycardia (148 beats per minute) with a prolonged QTc (554 ms) and ST-depressions in II, V2–V5 and ST-elevation in Avr, with normal R-wave progression. The initial laboratory results are depicted in Table 1.

Table 1. Laboratory results (No indication for follow-up or previously normalized).

	Day 1	Day 2	Reference Values
Hb (mmol/L)	12.5	10	8.5–11
Leucocytes (X 10^9/L)	34.4	27.9	4.0–10.0
Sodium (mmol/L)	142	140	135–147
Potassium (mmol/L)	2.6	3.9	3.5–5.0
Phosphate (mmol/L	0.53	0.66	0.70–1.50
Magnesium (mmol/L)	0.68	0.87	0.70–1.00
Glucose (mmol/L)	11.6	6.8	4.0–7.8
Creatinine (umol/L)	137	75	59–104
AST (U/L)	42	-	<35
ALT (U/L)	92	-	<45
Creatine kinase (U/L)	483	-	<171
pH	7.55	7.51	7.35–7.45
Bicarbonate (mmol/L)	21.1	22.4	22.0–29.0
Lactate (mmol/L)	5.0	1.7	0.5–1.7
CK-MB (ug/L)	16	-	<7.6
Hs-trop T (ug/L)	0.066	-	<0.014

Hb: haemoglobin, AST: aspartate transaminase, ALT: alanine transaminase, CK-MB: creatine kinase-myocardial band, HS-trop T: high-sensitive troponin T.

Despite the presence of lactate acidosis, arterial blood gas analysis showed metabolic alkalemia due to continuous vomiting. The drugs-of-abuse toxicology screening in a urine sample (Quidel, Tox Drug Screen, 94600) was found positive for benzodiazepines and cocaine. The positive benzodiazepine screening was attributable to midazolam administered in the ambulance. Cocaine and benzoylecgonine (a metabolite of cocaine) were not detectable in serum via liquid chromatography coupled with multistage accurate mass spectrometry (LC-MS^n) and were therefore not clinically relevant. Initial treatment included infusion of isotonic liquids, electrolyte supplementation, and anti-emetics (including dexamethasone 12 mg). Despite supportive therapy, tachypnoea increased (40 breaths per minute), and the temperature rose to a fever (38.7 °C), in addition to persisting nausea, tachycardia and hypertension. Subsequently, the patient was admitted to the intensive care unit, where benzodiazepines and a continuous infusion of labetalol were initiated to treat anxiety and excesses in haemodynamics, respectively. In addition, CVVHD was initiated to increase caffeine elimination, using the MultifiltratePRO (Fresenius medical care) with an ultraflux AV1000S filter and regional citrate anticoagulation. The dialysate flow rate was set at 2 L/h and the blood flow rate at 100 mL/min at a temperature of 37 °C. Within three hours after initiating CVVHD, the fever resolved due to active cooling. Tachypnoea started declining some hours later. The follow-up of elevated cardiac blood markers showed a decrease six hours later. After 15 h of CVVHD, the patient's haemodynamics normalized. Therefore, labetalol could be withdrawn, and CVVHD was discontinued. Caffeine blood levels were taken at presentation, during CVVHD treatment and after completion of therapy, and are depicted in Figure 1. The caffeine serum concentration upon presentation was 70 mg/L and had dropped to 21 mg/L after CVVHD treatment. Using the therapeutic drug-management application MwPharm version 1.8.2.20 (Mediware), we were able to simulate the serum caffeine concentrations (see Figure 1 and Table 2) [11]. After 30 h of ICU admission, the patient was discharged to the internal medicine ward with telemetric monitoring of the heart rhythm and discharged home the next day.

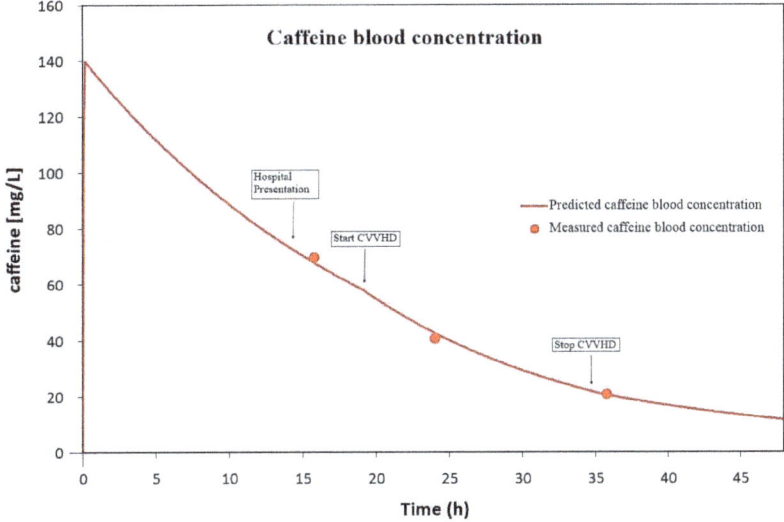

Figure 1. Caffeine blood concentration based on three caffeine blood samples extrapolated in a pharmacokinetic model using a therapeutic drug-management application.

Table 2. Pharmacokinetic parameters of caffeine blood concentration model.

Parameter	Population Value	Individual Value
Unbound fraction	0.64	0.64
Distribution volume	0.61 L/kg	0.86 (non-Bayesian) L/kg
Elimination constant	0.136 h^{-1}	0.0462 h^{-1}
Bioavailability	1	1
Absorption constant	19.8 h^{-1}	19.8 h^{-1}

3. Discussion

Despite the increasing popularity of energy drinks, most deaths resulting from caffeine overdose can be attributed to the consumption of diet pills and stimulants [12]. Initial symptoms of intoxication include nausea, vomiting, tachycardia, hypertension, hypotension, and convulsions. Secondary hypokalaemia, hyperglycaemia, hypocalcaemia, lactate acidosis, and rhabdomyolysis with subsequent kidney failure have been described. These biochemical changes and an increased sympathetic activity can result in cardiovascular complications, including potentially lethal arrhythmia and myocardial infarction [2,13,14]. Therapy includes preventing systemic absorption through gastric lavage and active charcoal combined with a laxative and should be initiated within 30–90 min after intake, based on caffeine's half-life time. However, since the half-life time can be prolonged in case of an overdose, active charcoal is possibly effective even after this period. Furthermore, therapy focuses on supportive care, such as electrolyte correction, fluid resuscitation, anti-emetics, beta-blockade and benzodiazepines, in the case of moderate to severe anxiety or convulsions [15]. These therapies require continuous monitoring of vital signs and biochemical markers. Therefore, admittance to a critical care unit is highly recommended in case of severe caffeine intoxication.

There are limited publications about using RRT in caffeine intoxication. Theophylline is also a xanthine derivate. It shows, structurally and in pharmacology, many similarities to caffeine. There are more publications about the use of RRT in theophylline intoxication. The EXtracorporeal TReatments In Poisoning workgroup (EXTRIP) published a guideline and recommended extracorporeal treatment in severe theophylline poisoning [16]. Clinical conditions can classify this severity (e.g., seizures or shock), as can a plasma concentration >100 mg/L. Intermittent haemodialysis is the preferred and recommended extracorporeal treatment, but hemoperfusion or CRRT (continuous renal replacement therapy), including CVVHD, are acceptable alternatives if haemodialysis is not available. In the article by Kim et al. [17], the authors provide a clear view on the differences between CRRT and haemodialysis in patients with an intoxication. The different extra-corporeal treatments are compared in the case of several well-known drug intoxications. The authors conclude that haemodialysis is the more effective treatment with all intoxications. The Dutch guidelines for intoxications agree with these conclusions but name CRRT as an acceptable suboptimal alternative [10]. The exceptions to this conclusion are patients who are haemodynamically unstable and in situations where haemodialysis is not available in the acute setting. Another indication for starting CRRT could be after the initial haemodialysis session to prevent a rebound rise of the drug. Although CRRT is less effective than haemodialysis, CRRT can be considered in intoxications with drugs that have a low protein binding, low volume of distribution (VD) and narrow therapeutic index. Examples of drugs where CRRT can be an acceptable alternative in intoxications are lithium, methanol and ethylene glycol.

The severity of intoxication, in this case, was based on the reported ingested amount and clinical presentation. Since death due to severe caffeine intoxication has been described after an oral intake of 5 g or more of caffeine [1,6], this patient's consumption of 10 g of caffeine was potentially lethal. Similarly, the predicted initial serum concentration was 140 mg/L, where concentrations of >80-100 mg/L are potentially lethal [2,8]. Based on the high ingested amount of caffeine, the high predicted blood levels, and the severity of the symptoms presented by our patient, we initiated CVVHD. Criteria for initiating haemodialysis in case of caffeine intoxication have been described by others [18]. The authors suggest that patients with severe clinical symptoms, in our case a tachycardia of >140 beats per minute, and high caffeine concentrations ≥140 mg/L can benefit from haemodialysis. Due to a delay in presentation, however, the initial serum concentration turned out to be 70 mg/L and did not therefore meet the suggested criteria. Even so, a concentration of 70 mg/L must still be considered a severe intoxication, since toxicity is seen at a caffeine serum concentration of >50 mg/L. The elevated initial serum concentration, even after a delay in presentation, illustrates the slow clearance of caffeine in case of an overdose. High serum caffeine concentrations result in the saturation of CYP1A2. Consequently, caffeine clearance follows non-linear kinetics in case of an overdose, thereby prolonging the half-life time from 5 h to >16 h, and up to 120 h has been described [2,3]. In this case, the half-life time was prolonged to 15 h (Figure 1), three times the half-life time of regular consumption. Due to this long half-life time, in combination with low VD and low plasma protein binding, toxin removal through CVVHD can be a valuable intervention to increase clearance and improve symptoms.

Caffeine concentrations can be quantified using immunoassays (ELISA) or high-performance liquid chromatography (HPLC). Even though ELISA may be more cost-effective, HPLC is the method of choice, since it has a high sensitivity and specificity [19,20]. In case of an intoxication, a high specificity is requested, since interference with other xanthine derivatives should be avoided. Sensitivity is less relevant, since intoxications generally concern high drug levels, which are measured to estimate the duration to a return to therapeutic drug levels and an indication for dialysis. Following the validated sensitivity and the high specificity of HPLC, we recommend HPLC as the quantification method of choice when used in the case of caffeine intoxication.

The effect of CVVHD is graphically illustrated in Figure 1, where the deflection in the curve at t = 19 h shows the additional effect of CVVHD in addition to the patient's clearance capacity. A more pronounced result can be expected using intermittent haemodialysis compared to CVVHD [3,21]. However, emergency haemodialysis is not always logistically possible or can be contra-indicated because of haemodynamic instability. We have shown that CVVHD can be a helpful alternative. Using high blood flow rates and high dialysis flow rates theoretically maximizes the effect of CVVHD on caffeine clearance; however, further studies are needed to test this hypothesis. Additionally, the effect of CVVHD can be more pronounced in the case of higher caffeine serum concentrations. Given caffeine's low plasma protein binding (17–36%), a higher plasma concentration will most likely lead to a higher percentage of unbound caffeine due to protein saturation. Since unbound caffeine is dialyzable, higher caffeine concentrations may result in additional serum clearance. Intermittent haemodialysis or CVVHD should therefore be reserved for cases involving severe, potentially lethal caffeine toxicity, hence with a high percentage of unbound caffeine. Additionally, a fast initiation of therapy will add to the effectiveness of CVVHD and therefore to its effectiveness in relation to symptoms of caffeine toxicity. We therefore stress the importance of an early recognition of caffeine toxicity. Once initiated, the duration of CVVHD therapy can best be adjusted to clinical response.

4. Conclusions

CVVHD may be an acceptable alternative to intermittent haemodialysis in the case of severe, potentially lethal caffeine intoxication, when intermittent haemodialysis is not available. Preferred treatment should always be haemodialysis, if possible. Overall CVVHD can be considered in intoxications with drugs that have low protein binding, low VD and a narrow therapeutic index. Adding Cytosorb could further improve effectivity. Both modalities should be reserved for cases of severe toxicity. Further research on the effect of higher blood flow rates may lead to a more effective use of CVVHD in case of caffeine intoxication.

Author Contributions: Conceptualization, E.J.R. and J.-W.H.J.G.; software, D.W.H.; validation, L.G.P., J.-W.H.J.G. and E.J.F.F.; investigation, E.J.R.; writing—original draft preparation, E.J.R. and D.W.H.; writing—review and editing, D.W.H., L.G.P. and J.-W.H.J.G.; supervision, J.-W.H.J.G. and E.J.F.F. All authors have read and agreed to the published version of the manuscript.

Funding: This research received no external funding.

Institutional Review Board Statement: Not applicable.

Informed Consent Statement: Written informed consent has been obtained from the patient to publish this paper.

Data Availability Statement: Not applicable.

Conflicts of Interest: The authors declare no conflict of interest.

References

1. Higdon, J.V.; Frei, B. Coffee and health: A review of recent human research. *Crit. Rev. Food Sci. Nutr.* **2006**, *46*, 101–123. [CrossRef] [PubMed]

2. Jaspers, T.C.C.; Ter Laak, M.; Kramers, C. *Toxicologie Behandelinformatie: Monografie Coffeïne*; Nationaal Vergiftigingen Informatie Centrum van het RIVM: Utrecht, The Netherlands, 2019.
3. Fausch, K.; Uehlinger, D.E.; Jakob, S.; Pasch, A. Haemodialysis in massive caffeine intoxication. *Clin. Kidney J.* **2012**, *5*, 150–152. [CrossRef] [PubMed]
4. Willson, C. The clinical toxicology of caffeine: A review and case study. *Toxicol. Rep.* **2018**, *5*, 1140–11452. [CrossRef] [PubMed]
5. Cappelletti, S.; Piacentino, D.; Sani, G.; Aromatario, M. Caffeine: Cognitive and physical performance enhancer or psychoactive drug? *Curr. Neuropharmacol.* **2015**, *13*, 71–88. [CrossRef] [PubMed]
6. Kerrigan, S.; Lindsey, T. Fatal caffeine overdose: Two case reports. *Forensic. Sci. Int.* **2005**, *153*, 67–69. [CrossRef] [PubMed]
7. Kromhout, H.E.; Landstra, A.M.; Van Luin, M.; Van Setten, P.A. Acute caffeine intoxication after intake of 'herbal energy capsules. *Ned. Tijdschr. Geneeskd.* **2008**, *152*, 1583–1586. [PubMed]
8. Cappelletti, S.; Piacentino, D.; Fineschi, V.; Frati, P.; Cipolloni, L.; Aromatario, M. Caffeine-Related Deaths: Manner of Deaths and Categories at Risk. *Nutrients* **2018**, *10*, 611. [CrossRef] [PubMed]
9. Gummin, D.D.; Mowry, J.B.; Beuhler, M.C.; Spyker, D.A.; Brooks, D.E.; Dibert, K.W.; Rivers, L.J.; Pham, N.; Ryan, M.L. 2019 Annual Report of the American Association of Poison Control Centers' National Poison Data System (NPDS): 37th Annual Report. *Clin. Toxicol.* **2020**, *58*, 1360–1541. [CrossRef] [PubMed]
10. Richtlijn Intoxicaties: Eerste opvang in het ziekenhuis. Federatie Medisch Specialisten. 2017. Available online: https://richtlijnendatabase.nl/richtlijn/intoxicaties_eerste_opvang_in_het_ziekenhuis/startpagina_intoxicaties.html (accessed on 4 February 2023).
11. Hardman, J.G.; Limbird, L.E.; Gilman, A.G. *Goodman & Gilman's the Pharmacological Basis of Therapeutics*, 10th ed.; McGraw-Hill: New York, NY, USA, 2001.
12. Temple, J.L.; Bernard, C.; Lipshultz, S.E.; Czachor, J.D.; Westphal, J.A.; Mestre, M.A. The Safety of Ingested Caffeine: A Comprehensive Review. *Front. Psychiatry* **2017**, *8*, 80. [CrossRef] [PubMed]
13. Andrade, A.; Sousa, C.; Pedro, M.; Fernandes, M. Dangerous mistake: An accidental caffeine overdose. *BMJ Case Rep.* **2018**, *2018*, bcr-2018-224185. [CrossRef] [PubMed]
14. Magdalan, J.; Zawadzki, M.; Skowronek, R.; Czuba, M.; Porębska, B.; Sozański, T.; Szpot, P. Nonfatal and fatal intoxications with pure caffeine-report of three different cases. *Forensic Sci. Med. Pathol.* **2017**, *13*, 355–358. [CrossRef] [PubMed]
15. Nationaal Vergiftigingen Informatie Centrum. Coffeine. UMC Utrecht; 2020 [updated 15-01-2020]. Available online: https://www.vergiftigingen.info/f?p=VI:PRINT:2859898901942:::1420:P1420_VERB_NO:6 (accessed on 16 December 2021).
16. Ghannoum, M.; Wiegand, T.J.; Liu, K.D.; Calello, D.P.; Godin, M.; Lavergne, V.; Gosselin, S.; Nolin, T.; Hoffman, R.S. Extracorporeal treatment for theophylline poisoning: Systematic review and recommendations from the EXTRIP workgroup. *Clin. Toxicol.* **2015**, *53*, 215–229. [CrossRef] [PubMed]
17. Kim, Z.; Goldfarb, D.S. Continuous renal replacement therapy does not have a clear role in the treatment of poisoning. *Nephron. Clin. Pract.* **2010**, *115*, c1-6. [CrossRef] [PubMed]
18. Yoshizawa, T.; Kamijo, Y.; Hanazawa, T.; Usui, K. Criterion for initiating hemodialysis based on serum caffeine concentration in treating severe caffeine poisoning. *Am. J. Emerg. Med.* **2021**, *46*, 70–73. [CrossRef] [PubMed]
19. Ohmichi, T.; Kasai, T.; Shinomoto, M.; Matsuura, J.; Koizumi, T.; Kitani-Morii, F.; Tatebe, H.; Sasaki, H.; Mizuno, T.; Tokuda, T. Quantification of Blood Caffeine Levels in Patients With Parkinson's Disease and Multiple System Atrophy by Caffeine ELISA. *Front. Neurol.* **2020**, *11*, 580127. [CrossRef] [PubMed]
20. Koller, D.; Vaitsekhovich, V.; Mba, C.; Steegmann, J.L.; Zubiaur, P.; Abad-Santos, F.; Wojnicz, A. Effective quantification of 11 tyrosine kinase inhibitors and caffeine in human plasma by validated LC-MS/MS method with potent phospholipids clean-up procedure. Application to therapeutic drug monitoring. *Talanta* **2020**, *208*, 120450. [CrossRef] [PubMed]
21. Ishigaki, S.; Fukasawa, H.; Kinoshita-Katahashi, N.; Yasuda, H.; Kumagai, H.; Furuya, R. Caffeine intoxication successfully treated by hemoperfusion and hemodialysis. *Intern. Med.* **2014**, *53*, 2745–2747. [CrossRef] [PubMed]

Disclaimer/Publisher's Note: The statements, opinions and data contained in all publications are solely those of the individual author(s) and contributor(s) and not of MDPI and/or the editor(s). MDPI and/or the editor(s) disclaim responsibility for any injury to people or property resulting from any ideas, methods, instructions or products referred to in the content.

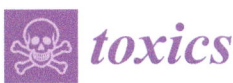

Case Report

Toxicological Analysis in Tissues Following Exhumation More Than Two Years after Death (948 Days): A Forensic Perspective in a Fatal Case

Giuseppe Davide Albano *, Stefania Zerbo, Corinne La Spina, Mauro Midiri, Daniela Guadagnino, Tommaso D'Anna, Roberto Buscemi and Antonina Argo

Section of Legal Medicine, Department of Health Promotion, Mother and Child Care, Internal Medicine and Medical Specialties, University of Palermo, 90129 Palermo, Italy
* Correspondence: giuseppedavide.albano@unipa.it

Abstract: Exhumations are performed in accordance with a court order and are crucial instruments in the investigation of death allegations. When a death is thought to be the result of drug misuse, pharmaceutical overdose, or pesticide poisoning, this process may be used on human remains. However, after a protracted postmortem interval (PMI), it might be difficult to detect the cause of death by looking at an exhumed corpse. The following case report reveals problems associated with postmortem drug concentration changes following exhumation more than two years after death. A 31-year-old man was found dead in a prison cell. On an inspection of the place, two blister packs, one with a tablet and the other empty, were taken and kept by the police officers. The evening before, the deceased would have taken cetirizine and food supplements consisting of carnitine–creatine tablets. No relevant autopsy findings have been observed. The toxicological analysis was performed by gas chromatography coupled to mass spectrometry and was negative for substances of abuse. Proteomic analysis was positive for creatine detection and negative for other drugs (clarithromycin, fenofibrate, and cetirizine). The presented case shows the methods, the findings, and the limitations of toxicological analysis in an exhumation case with a long postmortem interval (PMI).

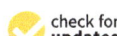

Citation: Albano, G.D.; Zerbo, S.; La Spina, C.; Midiri, M.; Guadagnino, D.; D'Anna, T.; Buscemi, R.; Argo, A. Toxicological Analysis in Tissues Following Exhumation More Than Two Years after Death (948 Days): A Forensic Perspective in a Fatal Case. *Toxics* **2023**, *11*, 485. https://doi.org/10.3390/toxics11060485

Academic Editor: Eric J. F. Franssen

Received: 31 March 2023
Revised: 19 May 2023
Accepted: 23 May 2023
Published: 26 May 2023

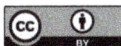

Copyright: © 2023 by the authors. Licensee MDPI, Basel, Switzerland. This article is an open access article distributed under the terms and conditions of the Creative Commons Attribution (CC BY) license (https://creativecommons.org/licenses/by/4.0/).

Keywords: exhumation; proteomic analysis; forensic; postmortem interval; sudden cardiac death

1. Introduction

An exhumation is an important tool in investigating suspicions of death, carried out under court order. It involves unburying a body, performing an autopsy, and evaluating all remains found near the body [1–4]. This procedure may be performed on human remains in the case of a death suspected to be due to poisoning with pesticides, medications, or drug abuse [3,5–8]. However, it can be challenging to diagnose by examining an exhumed corpse after a prolonged PMI. It may be difficult to differentiate actual lesions from autolytic changes, which should be carefully assessed. Moreover, postmortem toxicology investigations on exhumed human remains are rare but a true challenge for both the pathologist and the forensic toxicologist. Some drugs' concentrations may be influenced by the activity of certain enzymes, even after death [9]. Moreover, autolysis may cause the release of exogenous compounds [10]. Bacteria metabolism may influence the toxicological analysis results by using particular drugs or metabolites as substrates [11]. Furthermore, redistribution after death is influenced by the postmortem interval, even in the post-sampling and storage periods [12,13]. Previous reports stated the issues and limitations of toxicological analysis in exhumation cases, highlighting that conventional biological matrices may not be available due to putrefaction processes and that different postmortem phenomena may contribute to the reliability of toxicological findings [14,15]. Therefore, toxicological analysis of exhumed human remains is still a significant challenge. In this case report, we report our forensic investigation experience of a death in prison for which toxicological investigations were requested two years after the death. Prior to an exhumation, the question usually arises whether presumed morphological or toxicological findings can be detected after certain postmortem intervals. The presented case shows the methods, the findings, and the limitations of toxicological analysis in exhumation cases with a long postmortem interval (PMI).

2. Case Report

2.1. Case History

This is the case of a 31-year-old man found dead in a prison cell. On an inspection of the place, two blister packs, one with a tablet and the other empty, were taken and kept by the police officers. The evening before, the deceased would have taken cetirizine and food supplements consisting of carnitine–creatine tablets. A study of the documentation revealed in the anamnesis the presence of exertional precordialgiaextra-systolic arrhythmic activity, isolated ventricular premature beats (BEV), gastritis, and papulo-pustular acne.

Following this first judicial inspection, an autopsy examination was ordered, and thecompetent judicial authority (J.A.) ordered the dismissal of the case. However, more than two years later (948 days), the defenders of the deceased's family argued that the drugs taken the night before would have influenced the death event. Therefore, it was deemed necessary to proceed with the exhumation of the body.Among the questions posed was the need to proceed with the sampling to verify the presence of the drugs resulting from the prescribed therapy.

2.2. Autopsy Findings

The autoptic examination showed a male subject's corpse, apparentlyof regular build, with indefinable somatic characteristics due to the advanced putrefactive phenomenon. When the clothes were removed, the signs of the previous autoptic activity were revealed, with resection of the skullcap and cutting of the trunk; overall, the body had an appearance tending toward corification in the head–neck district, with a great representation of the putrefactive changes in the remaining part of the human residues of the exhumed body. The following organs were recognizable: stomach, intestine, aortic tract, and kidney; the state of decomposition made their removal superfluous for subsequent histopathological evaluations. The following tissues were collected and sampled for toxicological investigations: hair matrices, quadriceps muscles of the right thigh, and tissue fragments of possible renal origin.

2.3. Toxicological Analysis for Proteins, Drugs and Substances of Abuse

The toxicological analysis was carried out via gas chromatographic analysis with a mass detector of the extracts, acids, and bases subjected to a derivatization process. The extraction was carried out on organic residue. About 1 g of organic material was taken and finely minced with a mechanical instrument. Then, 4 mLof distilled water was added, and the whole was left to macerate for 48 h at 4 °C.

The sample was reconditioned at room temperature. It was then stirred on a rotating stirrer for 20′ and centrifuged for 10′ at 3500 rpm; the analysis was performed on the supernatants loaded on SPE cartridges bondelut certify Agilent 130 mg.The elution was performed with 2 mL of a freshly prepared mixture of dichloromethane and isopropanol containing 2% ammonia in a ratio of 78/20/2. The eluate was collected in a glass test tube containing 50 µLof a methanol/HCl mixture (9:1). The internal standard, i.e., a solution of the deuterated compounds, was added to the eluate before it dried.

The analysis was performed by gas chromatography technique coupled to mass spectrometry using an Agilent model 6890 N gas chromatograph connected to a model 5973 mass spectrometer operating at 70 eV with a source temperature of 230 °C; the instrument was operated using computers and Mass Hunter software.

An Agilent (Agilent Technologies Inc., Santa Clara, CA, USA) J&W DB-5 ms Ultra Inert capillary column with a length of 30 m, an internal diameter of 0.25 mm, and a film thickness of 0.25 µm was used for the chromatographic separation. The analysis was conducted with a programmed temperature starting from 150 °C for 1.00 min; then, the oven temperature was increased by 20 °C per minute up to 210 °C and maintained for 10 s; subsequently, the temperature was increasedfrom 20 °C by 10 °C per minute to reach the temperature of 250 °C, which was held for one minute. Finally, with a rise of 20 °C per minute, the temperature of 280 °C was reached and maintained for two minutes.The chromatographic run had a total duration of 11.2 min, and the data were acquired in sim (selected ion monitoring) mode. With the GC/MS technique, the identification of the substances present in the extracts occurred through the evaluation of the retention time of the gas chromatographic peak and its fragmentation spectrum; the latter was compared with those included in the computerized libraries with which the management software was equipped of the tool. Toxicological analyses were negative for substances of abuse and cetirizine presence. Analysis of the composition of food supplements (AMCO)for food products and supplements provides the hypothetical identity of the compounds present in the sample. Identification was made using the official database of the National Institute for Standards and Technologies (NIST) without the aid of a certified analytical standard. The test should be interpreted as a first-level screening. The detection of compounds is subject to the limits of instrumental detection.

The sample was digested using trypsin. An analysis was conducted in the auto-fragmentation acquisition mode. The data obtained were processed using SANIST Hb software with a generic "Uniprot" database. The results of this processingwere sent once the software had finished. An analysis was performed on thesample by looking for the compounds: creatine 132.13, detected; clarithromycin 748.47, not detected; and fenofibrate 361.11, not detected.

The sample was treated by enzymatic digestion with trypsin and analyzed in Auto Ms(n) acquisition mode. The data obtained were processed with the SANIST Hb software using a generic "Uniprot" database. From this processing, results were obtained with a statistical score of less than 30.

The sample was treated by enzymatic digestion with trypsin and analyzed in Auto Ms(n) acquisition mode. The data obtained were processed with the SANIST Hb software using a generic "Uniprot"database. From this processing, results were obtained with a statistical score of less than 30.

3. Discussion

In the specific case, the evening before the death, the patient had taken only one tablet of cetirizine and food supplements consisting of carnitine–creatine tablets. A single dose of carnitine can hardly reach a concentration to determine effects on cardiac repolarization, as in cases after prolonged administration, which can be evaluated by continuous activity on the QTC.

Indeed, the drug is well absorbed by the gastrointestinal tract after oral administration. The drug is distributed to biological tissues, reaching maximum plasma concentrations within one hour. The half-life of the drug is around 8 h. Cetirizine crosses the blood–brain barrier with difficulty, which accounts for the drug's minor sedative effects compared to other antihistamines. Plasma protein binding is 93%. Cetirizine is metabolized in the liver to a minimal extent and is an inactive metabolite. Elimination occurs by the renal route, with 60–70% of the drug eliminated in 24 h. A further 10% is excreted in the urine over 96 h. Reduced renal or hepatic function may result in slower elimination by prolonging its half-life. Half-life (T/2) is the time required for the amount of a drug in the body to decrease by 50% during elimination. Therefore, knowledge of the half-life of a drug is essential to allow adequate administration and avoid incurring an overdose. The half-life is a value independent of the drug's concentration and our body's metabolic activity. If the T/2 is short, then the decrease in concentration will be fast; conversely, the longer the half-life, the slighter the reduction in concentration. In daily clinical practice, the half-life is necessary to reach a specific effective plasma concentration value or to maintain a particular concentration of the plasma value of the drug for a long time (days or months) [16].

Therefore, it was assumed that after eight hours, the concentration of the drug was reduced by half, corresponding to 04.00–06.00 in the morning, the time of death, and still could not reach a stable concentration, which requires further administration over time. Therefore, it is difficult to assume that the single administered dose could have exerted such a pharmacological activity to alter the QTc and cause potential arrhythmia [17,18].

As for the carnitine and the creatine taken in the evening, it is noted that they are supplements (drugs) without adverse effects on the cardiovascular system, so much so that they are suggested as prophylactic protection in subjects receiving chemotherapy. In addition, when taken in high doses, it provides cardioprotection. In a review, the optimal amount was around 3g/day, with patients not obtaining better results even with higher doses of up to 6 g/day. Understood in the meaning of "drug," it has almost no contraindications and nearly no side effects, so much so that it is used as an over-the-counter drug, while its use as a supplement is as an anti-fatigue [5,11,19]. Carnitine is an endogenous product; however, in this case presentation, it was suspected by parents (irrespective of well-known scientific evidence) of ingestion as a protein-enriched food, which could interfere with the cardiac function of the dead man in jail. The prosecutor's office asked for such an analysis.

The above-described analysis of the literature on the incidence and the potential lethality of the patient's arrhythmic disturbances suggests the probable hypothesis that the patient's death was caused by a malignant ventricular arrhythmic event. The event was probably caused by a pre-existing extra-systolic focus of possible genetic nature and is still not always identifiable, as well as being a potential genetic character not detectable in ECG analysis [20–22].

To date, the toxicological investigations carried out have not allowed the detection of substances referred to in the pharmacological anamnesis. This outcome must, in any case, be evaluated in the context of studies carried out on widely degraded tissue samples of muscle matrix more than three years after the death and the sampling itself, making this investigation very limited in the reliability of the laboratory data.

In every test, choosing a practical sample type is an important choice. It is crucial to choose the right procedure if you want results that are legitimate and satisfying. The selection process is most strongly influenced by how valuable each sample type is [22,23].

When the analytes and sample matrix are defined, the next step is to develop a chromatographic system providing highly efficient separation for the targeted analytes and the corresponding matrix [24].

These techniques range from the simplest and currently rarely used, thin-layer chromatography (TLC), to capillary electrophoresis (CE) techniques, gas chromatography (GC), high-performance liquid chromatography (HPLC), and, finally, the most sophisticated, ultra-high-performance liquid chromatography (UHPLC) [25,26].

Substrates in postmortem toxicology are often seriously influenced by post-mortal degradation, redistribution, matrix effects, temperature, etc. Therefore, interpretation of the results may be difficult, especially when toxicological examinations must be carried out following exhumation. Many issues with various elements of decomposition may arise during the study of postmortem material. First, redistribution of many medications and poisons is known to happen throughout autolysis and into the putrefactive stage of decomposition, where residual enzyme activity can continue to metabolize pharmaceuticals and poisons. During putrefaction, bacteria that enter the body break down the tissues. The ensuing matrix of protein and lipid breakdown products can make it challenging to identify and quantify analytes. The same bacteria that putrefy the body can also break down medications and toxins inside the body, altering concentrations and perhaps causing the full loss of some analytes. Several of these drug breakdown pathways and their byproducts remain unknown. Recent studies suggest a possible role for metabolomics and proteomics in forensics to provide information about the assumption of substances and the postmortem interval. However, strong evidence is still lacking, and future research is needed to validate these methodologies and their application in the forensic field [27,28]. In the literature, comprehensive lists have been published called "expectation catalogues" on morphological and toxicological findings in relation to the postmortem interval. For this reason and due to the huge variety of possible issues, it may be difficult or impossible for even an experienced forensic specialist to acquire the necessary knowledge on his own [6–8,29–32] (Box 1).

Box 1. Take-home messages of toxicological and proteomic analysis in cases of autopsy tissues coming from exhumation with a high postmortem interval.

> **Key points**
> 1. A number of drugs are unstable either chemically (from pH changes), biochemically (from residual enzyme activity), or from use as substrates by putrefactive bacteria, or a combination of the above;
> 2. Postmortem redistribution of drugs and poisons increases with the postmortem interval, and peripheral blood samples should be analyzed in preference to those from central areas for quantitative purposes;
> 3. Byproducts of decomposition are putrefactive compounds, which can interfere with the analysis of drugs, particularly with less selective detectors;
> 4. The samples most frequently used in cases of toxicological investigations after exhumation with large PMI are: blood/plasma, hair, liver, and brain;
> 5. The most commonly used toxicological analysis techniques in cases of toxicological investigations after exhumation with large PMI are: thin-layer chromatography (TLC), capillary electrophoresis (CE) techniques, gas chromatography (GC), high performance liquid chromatography (HPLC), and finally, the most sophisticated, ultra-high-performance liquid chromatography (UHPLC);
> 6. Care should, therefore, be taken when interpreting quantitative drug and poison results in forensic toxicology, especially where there is evidence of putrefaction.

4. Conclusions

The toxicological investigations carried out did not allow the detection of substances referred to in the pharmacological anamnesis. The creatine detection was not relevant to the cause of death. This outcome must, in any case, be evaluated in the context of investigations carried out on tissue samples (largely degraded tissue fragments, mostly of the muscle matrix) taken more than two years after death, making this investigation very limited in the reliability of the laboratory data. Despite the great potential shown by these techniques, their active implementation in forensic investigations requires thorough validation studies to provide a uniform and certain interpretation of the results and strong reliability when the data are presented in a courtroom.

Author Contributions: Conceptualization, G.D.A., S.Z. and A.A.; methodology, A.A. and S.Z.; validation, S.Z., C.L.S. and A.A.; formal analysis, M.M., T.D., D.G. and R.B. investigation, R.B. and M.M.; resources, A.A.; data curation, C.L.S. and D.G. and T.D.; writing—original draft preparation, G.D.A. and C.L.S.; writing—review and editing, A.A. and S.Z.; visualization, M.M., D.G., T.D. and R.B.; supervision, S.Z. and A.A. All authors have read and agreed to the published version of the manuscript.

Funding: Supported Grant by University of Palermo, Eurostart 2021–22, cod. n. PRJ-1030. Title: "Tissue markers predictive of damage from substances of abuse and their correlation to preventable adverse cardiovascular events".

Institutional Review Board Statement: The manuscript describes a series of human studies performed in charge of Prosecutor Office for Forensic purposes; therefore, Ethics Committee or Institutional Review Board approval was not required. All procedures performed in this study were in accordance with the ethical standards of the institution and with the 1964 Helsinki Declaration and its later amendments or comparable ethical standards.

Informed Consent Statement: Informed consent was obtained from the relatives by Prosecutor Office.

Data Availability Statement: All data are included in the main text.

Conflicts of Interest: The authors declare no conflict of interest.

References

1. Ferllini, R. Tissue preservation and projectile context in a Spanish Civil War victim. *J. Forensic Leg. Med.* **2010**, *17*, 285–288. [CrossRef] [PubMed]
2. Fiedler, S.; Breuer, J.; Pusch, C.M.; Holley, S.; Wahl, J.; Ingwersen, J. Graveyards—Special landfills. *Sci. Total Environ.* **2012**, *419*, 90–97. [CrossRef] [PubMed]
3. Grellner, W.; Glenewinkel, F. Exhumations: Synopsis of morphological and toxicological findings in relation to the postmortem interval: Survey on a 20-year period and review of the literature. *Forensic Sci. Int.* **1997**, *90*, 139–159. [CrossRef] [PubMed]
4. Mirza, F.H.; Adil, S.E.; Memon, A.A.; Ali Paryar, H. Exhumation—Nuisance to the dead, justified? *J. Forensic Leg. Med.* **2012**, *19*, 337–340. [CrossRef]
5. Ehrlich, E.; Riesselmann, B.; Tsokos, M. A series of hospital homicides. *Leg. Med.* **2009**, *11*, S100–S102. [CrossRef]
6. Kaferstein, H.; Sticht, G.; Madea, B. Chlorprothixene in bodies after exhumation. *Forensic Sci. Int.* **2013**, *229*, e30–e34. [CrossRef]
7. Kumar, L.; Agarwal, S.S.; Chavali, K.H.; Mestri, S.C. Homicide by organophosphorus compound poisoning: A case report. *Med. Sci. Law* **2009**, *49*, 136–138. [CrossRef]
8. Spiller, H.A.; Pfiefer, E. Two fatal cases of selenium toxicity. *Forensic Sci. Int.* **2007**, *171*, 67–72. [CrossRef]
9. Evans, W.E.D. *The Chemistry of Death*; Charles C Thomas Publisher: Springfield, IL, USA, 1963.
10. Yarema, M.C.; Becker, C.E. Key concepts in postmortem drug redistribution. *Clin.Toxicol.* **2005**, *43*, 235–241. [CrossRef]
11. Robertson, M.; Drummer, O. Postmortem drug metabolism by bacteria. *J. Forensic Sci.* **1995**, *40*, 382–386. [CrossRef]
12. Pounder, D.J.; Jones, G.R. Post-mortem drug redistribution—A toxicological nightmare. *Forensic Sci. Int.* **1990**, *45*, 253–263. [CrossRef]
13. Paterson, S. Drugs and Decomposition. *Med. Sci. Law* **1993**, *33*, 103–109. [CrossRef]
14. Willeman, T.; Allibe, N.; Sauerbach, L.; Barret, A.; Eysseric-Guerin, H.; Paysant, F.; Stanke-Labesque, F.; Scolan, V. Homicidal poisoning series in a nursing home: Retrospective toxicological investigations in bone marrow and hair. *Int. J. Leg. Med.* **2021**, *136*, 123–131. [CrossRef]
15. Aknouche, F.; Ameline, A.; Kernalleguen, A.; Arbouche, N.; Maruejouls, C.; Kintz, P. Toxicological Investigations in a Death Involving 2,5-Dimethoxy-4-Chloamphetamine (DOC) Performed on an Exhumed Body. *J. Anal. Toxicol.* **2020**, *45*, e1–e7. [CrossRef]
16. Grumetto, L.; Cennamo, G.; Del Prete, A.; La Rotonda, M.I.; Barbato, F. Pharmacokinetics of cetirizine in tearfluid after a single oral dose. *Clin.Pharmacokinet.* **2002**, *41*, 525–531. [CrossRef]
17. Wadhwa, R.R.; Cascella, M. *Steady State Concentration*; StatPearls: Tampa, FL, USA, 2021.
18. Argo, A.; Zerbo, S.; Buscemi, R.; Trignano, C.; Bertol, E.; Albano, G.D.; Vaiano, F. A Forensic Diagnostic Algorithm for Drug-Related Deaths: A Case Series. *Toxics* **2022**, *10*, 152. [CrossRef]
19. Shang, R.; Sun, Z.; Li, H. Effective dosing of L-carnitine in the secondary prevention of cardiovascular disease: A systematic review and meta-analysis. *BMC Cardiovasc. Disord.* **2014**, *14*, 88. [CrossRef]
20. Bertol, E.; Vaiano, F.; Argo, A.; Zerbo, S.; Trignano, C.; Protani, S.; Favretto, D. Overdose of Quetiapine—A Case Report with QT Prolongation. *Toxics* **2021**, *9*, 339. [CrossRef]
21. Zerbo, S.; Lanzarone, A.; Raimondi, M.; Martino, L.D.; Malta, G.; Cappello, F.; Argo, A. Myocardial bridge pathology and preventable accidents during physical activity of healthy subjects: A case report and a literature review. *Med.-Leg. J.* **2020**, *88*, 209–214. [CrossRef]
22. Argo, A.; Sortino, C.; Zerbo, S.; Averna, L.; Procaccianti, P. Sudden unexplained juvenile death and the role of medicolegal investigation: Update on molecular autopsy. *EuroMediterr. Biomed. J.* **2012**, *145*, 7.
23. Castillo-Peinado, L.; de Castro, M.L. Present and foreseeable future of metabolomics in forensic analysis. *Anal. Chim. Acta* **2016**, *925*, 1–15. [CrossRef] [PubMed]
24. Gonzalez-Riano, C.; Garcia, A.; Barbas, C. Metabolomics studies in brain tissue: A review. *J. Pharm. Biomed. Anal.* **2016**, *130*, 141–168. [CrossRef] [PubMed]
25. Milman, B. Techniques and Methods of Identification. In *Chemical Identification and Its Quality Assurance*; Springer: Berlin/Heidelberg, Germany, 2011; Volume 18, pp. 23–39.
26. Zhang, Y.V.; Wei, B.; Zhu, Y.; Zhang, Y.; Bluth, M.H. Liquid Chromatography-Tandem Mass Spectrometry: An Emerging Technology in the Toxicology Laboratory. *Clin. Lab. Med.* **2016**, *36*, 635–661. [CrossRef] [PubMed]
27. Mok, J.-H.; Joo, M.; Duong, V.-A.; Cho, S.; Park, J.-M.; Eom, Y.-S.; Song, T.-H.; Lim, H.-J.; Lee, H. Proteomic and Metabolomic Analyses of Maggots in Porcine Corpses for Post-Mortem Interval Estimation. *Appl. Sci.* **2021**, *11*, 7885. [CrossRef]
28. Duong, V.A.; Park, J.M.; Lim, H.J.; Lee, H. Proteomics in forensic analysis: Applications for human samples. *Appl. Sci.* **2021**, *11*, 3393. [CrossRef]
29. Althoff, H. Bei welchen Fragestellungen kann man aussagefahige pathomorphologische Befunde nach Exhumierung erwarten? *Z. Rechtsmed.* **1974**, *75*, 1–20. [CrossRef]
30. Spennemann, D.H.; Franke, B. Archaeological techniques for exhumations: A unique data source for crime scene investigations. *Forensic Sci. Int.* **1995**, *74*, 5–15. [CrossRef]

31. Albano, G.D.; Malta, G.; La Spina, C.; Rifiorito, A.; Provenzano, V.; Triolo, V.; Vaiano, F.; Bertol, E.; Argo, A. Toxicological Findings of Self-Poisoning Suicidal Deaths: A Systematic Review by Countries. *Toxics* **2022**, *10*, 654. [CrossRef]
32. Triolo, V.; Spanò, M.; Buscemi, R.; Gioè, S.; Malta, G.; Čaplinskiene, M.; Argo, A. EtG Quantification in Hair and Different Reference Cut-Offs in Relation to Various Pathologies: A Scoping Review. *Toxics* **2022**, *10*, 682. [CrossRef]

Disclaimer/Publisher's Note: The statements, opinions and data contained in all publications are solely those of the individual author(s) and contributor(s) and not of MDPI and/or the editor(s). MDPI and/or the editor(s) disclaim responsibility for any injury to people or property resulting from any ideas, methods, instructions or products referred to in the content.

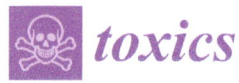

Case Report

Internet-Purchased Sodium Azide Used in a Fatal Suicide Attempt: A Case Report and Review of the Literature

Lisa T. van der Heijden [1,2,*], Karen E. van den Hondel [3], Erik J. H. Olyslager [4], Lutea A. A. de Jong [4], Udo J. L. Reijnders [3] and Eric J. F. Franssen [5]

1. Department of Pharmacy & Pharmacology, Antoni van Leeuwenhoek/The Netherlands Cancer Institute, 1066 CX Amsterdam, The Netherlands
2. Division of Pharmacology, Antoni van Leeuwenhoek/The Netherlands Cancer Institute, 1066 CX Amsterdam, The Netherlands
3. Department of Forensic Medicine, GGD Amsterdam, 1066 CX Amsterdam, The Netherlands
4. Department of Clinical Pharmacy, Expert Center Gelre-iLab, Gelre Hospitals, 1066 CX Apeldoorn/Zutphen, The Netherlands
5. Department of Clinical Pharmacy, OLVG Hospital, 1066 CX Amsterdam, The Netherlands; e.j.f.franssen@olvg.nl
* Correspondence: l.vd.heijden@nki.nl; Tel.: +31-020-512-7928

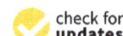

Citation: van der Heijden, L.T.; van den Hondel, K.E.; Olyslager, E.J.H.; de Jong, L.A.A.; Reijnders, U.J.L.; Franssen, E.J.F. Internet-Purchased Sodium Azide Used in a Fatal Suicide Attempt: A Case Report and Review of the Literature. *Toxics* **2023**, *11*, 608. https://doi.org/10.3390/toxics11070608

Academic Editor: Guido Cavaletti

Received: 13 June 2023
Revised: 6 July 2023
Accepted: 11 July 2023
Published: 13 July 2023

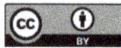

Copyright: © 2023 by the authors. Licensee MDPI, Basel, Switzerland. This article is an open access article distributed under the terms and conditions of the Creative Commons Attribution (CC BY) license (https:// creativecommons.org/licenses/by/ 4.0/).

Abstract: There has been a significant increase in sodium azide intoxications since the 1980s. Intoxications caused by sodium azide are becoming increasingly prevalent in the Netherlands as a result of its promotion for the purpose of self-euthanasia. The mechanism of toxicity is not completely understood but is dose-dependent. The presented case describes a suicide by sodium azide of a young woman (26 years old) with a history of depression and suicide attempts. The decedent was found in the presence of prescription medicine, including temazepam, domperidone in combination with omeprazole, and the chemical preservative sodium azide. Quantitative toxicology screening of whole blood revealed the presence of 70 μg/L temazepam (toxic range > 1000 μg/L) and 28 mg/L sodium azide (fatal range: 2.6–262 mg/L). Whole blood qualitative analysis revealed the presence of temazepam, temazepam-glucuronide, olanzapine, n-desmethylolanzapine, and acetaminophen. In circles promoting sodium azide, it is recommended to use sodium azide in combination with medications targeting sodium azide's negative effects, such as analgesics, antiemetics, and anti-anxiety drugs. The medicines recovered at the body's location, as well as the results of the toxicology screens, were consistent with the recommendations of self-euthanasia using sodium azide.

Keywords: sodium azide; postmortem toxicology; suicide

1. Introduction

Sodium azide (NaN_3) is the conjugate base of hydrazoic acid (HN_3) [1]. It is a white crystalline powder that is tasteless, odorless, and highly soluble in water [1]. Sodium azide transforms into hydrazoic acid when it comes into contact with water [1,2]. The compound is used in several fields, most notably as a propellant in vehicular airbags and safety chutes in airplanes [3]. Other applications of sodium azide are as a facilitator in synthetic reactions in chemical laboratories and as a preservative to inhibit microbial growth in biomedical laboratories [4].

In recent years, there has been a rise in the number of reports detailing (deadly) poisonings caused by sodium azide. Since the 1980s, there has been a significant increase in sodium azide intoxications in comparison to previous decades [2]. Continuing, there has been an increase in the number of suicides committed with sodium azide since the year 2000 [2]. In 2021, 37% of all case reports regarding sodium azide intoxications were suicide attempts [2]. The fatality of a sodium azide intoxication is approximately 50%, but increases to 92% if only suicide attempts are taken into account [2]. As a result of sodium azide's promotion as a substance for use in self-euthanasia, the incidence of sodium azide poisonings increased in the Netherlands and surrounding countries [5,6]. It is likely that the convenience of purchasing the substance through online retailers has contributed to the increase in the usage of sodium azide as a (fatal) method of suicide [7,8].

The mechanism of toxicity of sodium azide is not completely elucidated. In the liver, sodium azide is metabolized to nitrogen oxide, which causes hypotension and arrhythmia [9,10]. In addition, sodium azide irreversibly blocks Cytochrome C oxidase by inhibiting oxidative phosphorylation, resulting in cell death [1]. Sodium azide also inhibits catalase, an enzyme responsible for the detoxification of hydrogen peroxide to water and oxygen [11], which can reduce ATP synthesis and cause oxidative stress [4]. The toxicity of sodium azide is dose-dependent [12]. Lower doses may result in nausea, vomiting, hypotension, tachycardia, and headaches, whereas higher doses can lead to prolonged hypotension, dysrhythmias, acidosis, seizures, and eventually death [13]. Lethal doses are reported to be above 700 mg or 10 mg/kg [14,15], while toxic doses are reported to be between 20 and 180 mg [15]. The average time between ingestion and death is 4.5 h [1].

The current case describes a suicide with sodium azide of a young woman with a history of depression and suicide attempts and illustrates the need for research of the epidemiology of sodium azide poisonings as well as ambiguous recommendations regarding toxicology screening.

2. Case Report

Early in the morning, a friend of the decedent (female, 26 years old), contacted the police after receiving an alarming text, which resembled a farewell message. The police arrived at the house of the decedent within an hour, finding several medications in the bedroom of the decedent. Several strips of temazepam 10 mg were discovered on the desk, although one of the strips was missing seven pills. In addition, there was half a strip of domperidone 10 mg on the desk, of which two tablets were missing, and a jar with omeprazole with the name of the decedent. On one of the desk's shelves, a white container with a white crystalline substance was discovered. According to the label, it contained 25 g of sodium azide. External examination was performed by a forensic physician in collaboration with crime scene technicians and detectives. In the Netherlands, external examinations are performed by a forensic physician in cases of suspected unnatural causes of death or when the general practitioner is unavailable or unknown [16]. While routine post-mortem toxicological screening has not been implemented in all regions of the Netherlands, the collection of urine and femoral blood for toxicology screening has become increasingly part of the medical examination. A forensic autopsy is only performed when the case report contains questions regarding the cause of death (suspected crime). Clinical autopsies are not commonly performed due to their costly and time-consuming procedures [16,17].

The decedent had a history of depression and schizophrenia and was previously hospitalized for 10 weeks in an institution for adults with severe psychiatric disorders or addiction. Continuing, the decedent received outpatient treatment. The decedent had few social contacts, most of which she kept over the internet. The decedent also had a history of suicide attempts, and, according to her mother, the decedent had talked about the use of sodium azide in the past and communicated that she had ordered the compound online.

Toxicology screening was performed on whole blood and urine. The femoral-collected NaF-preserved blood sample was stored at $-20\ °C$ until analysis. Qualitative analysis of the whole blood sample revealed the presence of temazepam, temazepam-glucuronide, olanzapine, n-desmethylolanzapine, and paracetamol. Domperidone and omeprazole were not part of the toxicology screening. Acetone, ethanol, isopropanol, and methanol were not present in the whole blood sample. Additional quantitative analysis was performed on the whole blood sample for temazepam and sodium azide using validated LC-MS/MS and GC-MS methods, respectively. Except for the highest QC for sodium azide, which demonstrated a 16.2% bias, the methods were linear, and showed a bias of $+/-15\%$ and a precision less than 15% throughout the entire measuring range. The temazepam blood concentration was 70 μg/L (toxic range > 1000 μg/L), and the sodium azide blood concentration was 28 mg/L, which was above the upper limit of quantification (10 mg/L). A sodium azide concentration of 28 mg/L falls within the range of reported fatal concentrations [15]. Lastly, the toxicology screening of the urine sample was only positive for benzodiazepines.

3. Discussion

This case report presents a fatal intoxication with sodium azide after obtaining the compound through an online retailer. Sodium azide has been promoted as a drug for self-euthanasia in the Netherlands since 2017 [18]. After the first news report about drugs for self-euthanasia, a retailer reported increased sales of sodium azide [19]. However, the incidence of self-euthanasia with sodium azide, or other self-euthanasia drugs, is unknown [18]. The "right-to-die" organization supporting sodium azide for self-euthanasia recommended the administration of 1–2 g of sodium azide, along with pain killers, antiemetics, and medications used for insomnia or anxiety [18]. In the current case report, the decedent was found in the presence of the antiemetic domperidone and temazepam. These findings suggest the decedent followed the recommendations regarding self-euthanasia with sodium azide. Furthermore, the whole blood samples collected from the decedent were positive for acetaminophen. While sodium azide is recommended as a quick and humane manner of self-euthanasia, the recommended co-medication and the described symptoms discredit this claim [4,11,12,18].

The use of sodium azide is hazardous because there is no antidote or effective therapy for sodium azide poisoning available. Sodium azide demonstrates similarities to cyanide poising. However, neither treatment with sodium thiosulfate nor treatment with sodium nitrite improves clinical outcomes [12,13,20]. There is a hypothesis that methylene blue may prevent seizures caused by sodium azide by scavenging nitric oxide in the brain [21,22]. However, to date, no cases have been reported in which methylene blue has been successfully used as an antidote. Other case reports described a variety of therapeutic supportive care interventions, including sodium thiosulfate, intralipid, gastric lavage with activated charcoal, hydroxocobalamin, dopamine, dobutamine, methylprednisolone, calcium gluconate, insulin/glucose, sodium bicarbonate, and adrenaline [4,14,23,24]. Despite extensive and aggressive supportive care measures such as exchange transfusion or dialysis, in addition to the above-described therapeutic strategies, all of these individuals had to be resuscitated, and all were unsuccessful [4,14,23,24]. However, it is suggested that there might be a window of opportunity for the use of exchange transfusions or dialysis if applied before systemic effects [4] and in patients with no severe hemodynamic symptoms [14]. Due to the rapid onset of symptoms after a (high) dose of sodium azide, this treatment window may be limited.

Quantitative analysis of the deceased's whole blood samples confirmed a sodium azide concentration of 28 mg/L, which is within the known range of fatal sodium azide concentrations (2.6–262 mg/L) [15]. In acute intoxications, the typical blood concentrations are around 50 mg/L [2]. The variability in reported sodium azide levels may be partially attributable to sodium azide's instability in post-mortem biological material [2]. In vitro, the half-life of azide was 2.5 days at ambient temperature and 12 days at 0 °C [25]. Sodium azide was stable for 49 days in whole blood stored at −20 °C [26,27] and 49 days in plasma at −20 °C and −70 °C [24]. Therefore, it is recommended to store biological samples at −20 °C or −70 °C, protected from light. Neutralizing the pH of the matrix is another method to improve the stability of sodium azide [26]. The current reported sodium azide blood concentration of 28 mg/L could possibly be an underestimation, since the sample was thawed when it was received at the location of analysis. A second factor that could contribute to the reported range of sodium azide levels is its fast elimination [24]. Sodium azide has a reported half-life of 2.5 h in living individuals and may be detected approximately 12 h after ingestion [28]. The rapid clearance of sodium azide is consistent with findings from a number of case reports in which sodium azide was not detectable in plasma or blood but was quantifiable in stomach content [24,27]. In this case report, blood sodium azide concentrations were quantifiable, which is consistent with the time between sample collection and the estimated time of death (approximately 5 h).

The above discussion addresses several subjects that should be investigated further. First, the epidemiology of sodium azide intoxications is incompletely understood and should be investigated further. The incidence of self-euthanasia with sodium azide and information about how people obtain the compound could inform preventative strategies and legislation (e.g., steps are being taken in the Netherlands to increase the difficulty for private individuals to obtain sodium azide). Moreover, unambiguous recommendations regarding toxicology screening for suspected sodium azide poisonings are necessary. Lastly, a better understanding of the toxicological mechanism of sodium azide is essential for more and better-informed treatment options.

4. Conclusions

The presented case describes a suicide of a young woman with a history of depression and suicidal behavior using sodium azide. The medications found at the location of the body and the results of the toxicological tests were consistent with the recommendations of self-euthanasia with sodium azide. There are indications in the literature that the commercial availability of sodium azide is hazardous. More research is needed regarding the epidemiology of sodium azide poisonings, and ambiguous recommendations regarding toxicology screening are desired.

Author Contributions: Conceptualization: L.T.v.d.H. and E.J.F.F.; Investigation: E.J.H.O.; Supervision: E.J.F.F.; Writing—original draft: L.T.v.d.H.; Writing—review & eiditing: K.E.v.d.H., E.J.H.O., L.A.A.d.J., U.J.L.R. and E.J.F.F. All authors have read and agreed to the published version of the manuscript.

Funding: This research received no external funding.

Data Availability Statement: Data available on request due to restrictions e.g., privacy or ethical.

Conflicts of Interest: The authors declare no conflict of interest.

References

1. Chang, S.; Lamm, S.H. Human Health Effects of Sodium Azide Exposure: A Literature Review and Analysis. *Int. J. Toxicol.* **2003**, *22*, 175–186. [CrossRef] [PubMed]
2. Wachełko, O.; Zawadzki, M.; Szpot, P. A novel procedure for stabilization of azide in biological samples and method for its determination (HS-GC-FID/FID). *Sci. Rep.* **2021**, *11*, 15568. [CrossRef] [PubMed]
3. Francis, D.; Warren, S.A.; Warner, K.J.; Harris, W.; Copass, M.K.; Bulger, E.M. Sodium Azide-Associated Laryngospasm After Air Bag Deployment. *J. Emerg. Med.* **2010**, *39*, e113–e115. [CrossRef] [PubMed]
4. Tat, J.; Heskett, K.; Satomi, S.; Pilz, R.B.; Golomb, B.A.; Boss, G.R. Sodium azide poisoning: A narrative review. *Clin. Toxicol.* **2021**, *59*, 683–697. [CrossRef]
5. Workum, J.D.; Bisschops, L.L.A.; van den Berg, M.J.W. Auto-intoxicatie met 'zelfmoordpoeder'. *Ned Tijdschr Geneeskd* **2019**, *163*, D3369.
6. Van Riel, A.J.; Wijnands-Kleukers, A.P.; Dekker, D.; De Vries, I.; De Lange, D.W. Death on demand: Public debate leads to increasing use of "suicide powders". *Clin. Toxicol.* **2019**, *57*, 539–540.
7. Holstege, C.P.; Bechtel, L.K.; Reilly, T.H.; Wispelwey, B.P.; Dobmeier, S.G. Unusual But Potential Agents of Terrorists. *Emerg. Med. Clin. N. Am.* **2007**, *25*, 549–566. [CrossRef]
8. Leonard, J.B.; Hines, E.Q.; Anderson, B.D. Prime eligible poisons: Identification of extremely hazardous substances available on Amazon.com®. *Clin. Toxicol.* **2019**, *58*, 45–48. [CrossRef]
9. Frawley, K.L.; Totoni, S.C.; Bae, Y.; Pearce, L.L.; Peterson, J. A Comparison of Potential Azide Antidotes in a Mouse Model. *Chem. Res. Toxicol.* **2020**, *33*, 594–603. [CrossRef] [PubMed]
10. Smith, R.P.; Louis, C.A.; Kruszyna, R.; Kruszyna, H. Acute neurotoxicity of sodium azide and nitric oxide*1. *Fundam. Appl. Toxicol.* **1991**, *17*, 120–127. [CrossRef]
11. Keilin, D.H.E. Inhibitors of catalase reaction. *Nature* **1934**, *134*, 933. [CrossRef]
12. Klein-Schwartz, W.; Gorman, R.L.; Oderda, G.M.; Massaro, B.P.; Kurt, T.L.; Garriott, J.C. Three Fatal Sodium Azide Poisonings. *Med. Toxicol. Advers. Drug Exp.* **1989**, *4*, 219–227. [CrossRef] [PubMed]

13. Schwarz, E.S.; Wax, P.M.; Kleinschmidt, K.C.; Sharma, K.; Chung, W.M.; Cantu, G.; Spargo, E.; Todd, E. Multiple Poisonings with Sodium Azide at a Local Restaurant. *J. Emerg. Med.* **2014**, *46*, 491–494. [CrossRef] [PubMed]
14. Groeneveld, N.A.; van Hoeven, L.; van der Crabben, R.; Uil, C.D.; Bethlehem, C.; Alsma, J. Potential therapies for sodium azide intoxication; a case report and review of the literature. *Acute Med. J.* **2022**, *21*, 86–95. [CrossRef]
15. Baselt, R.C. *Disposition of Toxic Drugs and Chemicals in Man*, 10th ed.; Biomedical Publications: Seal Beach, CA, USA, 2014.
16. Bisch, A.; Ceelen, M.; Dorn, T.; Reijnders, U.; Hondel, K.V.D.; Stomp, J.; Burger, J.D.; Franssen, E. Performance of an on-site urine multidrug test used by forensic physicians in determining the cause of death. *J. Forensic Leg. Med.* **2022**, *88*, 102346. [CrossRef]
17. De Groot, R.; Van Zoelen, G.A.; Leenders, M.E.C.; Van Riel, A.J.H.P.; De Vries, I.; De Lange, D.W. Is secondary chemical exposure of hospital personnel of clinical importance? *Clin. Toxicol.* **2021**, *59*, 269–278. [CrossRef]
18. Braam, S. De opkomst en ondergang van 'middel X'. *Ned Tijdschr Geneeskd* **2019**, 163.
19. Goossen, H. *Bestellingen Voor 'Ethanasiapoeder' bij Beeks Bdrijf*; De Limburger: Limburg, The Netherlands, 2017.
20. Emmett, E.A.; Ricking, J.A. Fatal Self-Administration of Sodium Azide. *Ann. Intern. Med.* **1975**, *83*, 224–226. [CrossRef]
21. Groeneveld, N.; van Hoeven, L.; Bethlehem, C.; Alsma, J. Comment on sodium azide poisoning. *Clin. Toxicol.* **2021**, *60*, 539–540. [CrossRef]
22. Abbanat, R.A.; Smith, R.P. The influence of methemoglobinemia on the lethality of some toxic anions: I. Azide. *Toxicol. Appl. Pharmacol.* **1964**, *6*, 576–583. [CrossRef] [PubMed]
23. Richardson, S.G.; Giles, C.; Swan, C.H. Two cases of sodium azide poisoning by accidental ingestion of Isoton. *J. Clin. Pathol.* **1975**, *28*, 350–351. [CrossRef]
24. Bruin, M.A.C.; Dekker, D.; Venekamp, N.; Tibben, M.; Rosing, H.; de Lange, D.W.; Beijnen, J.H.; Huitema, A.D.R. Toxicological analysis of azide and cyanide for azide intoxications using gas chromatography. *Basic Clin. Pharmacol. Toxicol.* **2020**, *128*, 534–541. [CrossRef] [PubMed]
25. Kruszyna, R.; Smith, R.P.; Kruszyna, H. Determining sodium azide concentration in blood by ion chromatography. *J. Forensic Sci.* **1998**, *43*, 200–202. [CrossRef] [PubMed]
26. Ohmori, T.; Ohsawa, I.; Komano, A.; Kishi, S.; Sato, T.; Seto, Y. High distribution of azide in blood investigated in vivo, and its stability in blood investigated in vitro. *Forensic Toxicol.* **2014**, *32*, 251–257. [CrossRef]
27. Le Blanc-Louvry, I.; Laburthe-Tolra, P.; Massol, V.; Papin, F.; Goullé, J.P.; Lachatre, G.; Gaulier, J.M.; Proust, B. Suicidal sodium azide intoxication: An analytical challenge based on a rare case. *Forensic Sci. Int.* **2012**, *221*, e17–e20. [CrossRef]
28. Senda, T.; Nishio, K.; Hori, Y.; Baba, A.; Suzuki, Y.; Asari, Y.; Tsuchimoto, K. A case of fatal acute sodium azide poisoning. *Chudoku Kenkyu* **2001**, *14*, 339–342.

Disclaimer/Publisher's Note: The statements, opinions and data contained in all publications are solely those of the individual author(s) and contributor(s) and not of MDPI and/or the editor(s). MDPI and/or the editor(s) disclaim responsibility for any injury to people or property resulting from any ideas, methods, instructions or products referred to in the content.

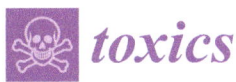

Case Report

Fatal Overdose with the Cannabinoid Receptor Agonists MDMB-4en-PINACA and 4F-ABUTINACA: A Case Report and Review of the Literature

Gábor Simon [1,*], Mónika Kuzma [1], Mátyás Mayer [1,2], Karola Petrus [1] and Dénes Tóth [1]

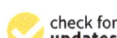

Citation: Simon, G.; Kuzma, M.; Mayer, M.; Petrus, K.; Tóth, D. Fatal Overdose with the Cannabinoid Receptor Agonists MDMB-4en-PINACA and 4F-ABUTINACA: A Case Report and Review of the Literature. *Toxics* **2023**, *11*, 673. https://doi.org/10.3390/toxics11080673

Academic Editor: Eric J. F. Franssen

Received: 24 June 2023
Revised: 2 August 2023
Accepted: 3 August 2023
Published: 5 August 2023

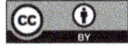

Copyright: © 2023 by the authors. Licensee MDPI, Basel, Switzerland. This article is an open access article distributed under the terms and conditions of the Creative Commons Attribution (CC BY) license (https:// creativecommons.org/licenses/by/ 4.0/).

[1] Department of Forensic Medicine, Medical School, University of Pécs, Szigeti str. 12, H-7624 Pécs, Hungary; monika.kuzma@aok.pte.hu (M.K.); matyas.mayer@aok.pte.hu (M.M.); karola.petrus@aok.pte.hu (K.P.); denes.toth@aok.pte.hu (D.T.)

[2] Department of Laboratory Medicine, Medical School, University of Pécs, Szigeti str. 12, H-7624 Pécs, Hungary

* Correspondence: gabor.simon@aok.pte.hu; Tel.: +36-72-536230

Abstract: A case of a 26-year-old male who died from consuming synthetic cannabinoid receptor agonists MDMB-4en-PINACA and 4F-ABUTINACA is reported. MDMB-4en-PINACA and 4F-ABUTINACA are potent synthetic cannabinoid receptor agonists (SCRAs). This is the first detailed reporting of MDMB-4-en-PINACA and 4F-ABUTINACA associated fatality, which can help the routine forensic work. The scientific literature on the symptoms associated with these substances are evaluated, along with the pharmacological properties and possible mechanism of death. A forensic autopsy was performed according to Recommendation No. R (99)3 of the Council of Europe on medico-legal autopsies. Histological samples were stained with hematoxylin and eosin (HE). Complement component C9 immunohistochemistry was applied to all heart samples. Toxicological analyses were carried out by supercritical fluid chromatography coupled with tandem mass spectrometry (SFC-MS/MS) and headspace gas chromatography with a flame ionization detector (HS-GC-FID). The literature was reviewed to identify reported cases of MDMB-4en-PINACA and 4F-ABUTINACA use. Autopsy findings included brain edema, internal congestion, petechial bleeding, pleural ecchymoses, and blood fluidity. Toxicological analyses determined 7.2 ng/mL of MDMB-4en-PINACA and 9.1 ng/mL of 4F-ABUTINACA in the peripheral blood. MDMB-4en-PINACA and 4F-ABUTINACA are strong, potentially lethal SCRA, and their exact effects and outcome are unpredictable.

Keywords: forensic pathology; forensic toxicology; synthetic cannabinoid; MDMB-4en-PINACA; 4F-ABUTINACA; overdose; autopsy

1. Introduction

Synthetic cannabinoid receptor agonists (SCRAs) first appeared as a legal alternative to cannabis in 2004, and they have been linked to numerous fatalities since then [1]. SCRAs have diverse toxicological effects, including renal injury (proximal tubular dilation and tubular necrosis), cardiotoxicity (arrhythmias, myocardial infarction, heart failure, cardiomyopathies), respiratory depression, gastrointestinal symptoms (abdominal pain, vomiting), epilepsy, and a broad spectrum of psychiatric symptoms [2–6]. SCRA toxicity can be related to fatalities directly (alone or mono intoxication), or indirectly (behavioral and physical contribution), but many times their contributory role is not clear [7,8]. The main problem with the forensic evaluation of potentially SCRA-related fatalities is that the concentration threshold that could be fatal is poorly defined and exhibits significant variations, especially in light of the several different SCRAs consumed [8]. Detailed reports—including autopsy findings and toxicological results—of fatal cases associated exclusively or partially with SCRAs (and other psychoactive substances) can be advised to help understand their mechanism of effect and establish potentially toxic and fatal concentrations for each substance, thus helping everyday forensic practice. It is especially important in the case of widely used compounds.

MDMB-4en-PINACA—also known as MDMB-PENINACA, 5Cl-ADB-A, or ADB-PINACA-A, with the IUPAC name methyl (S)-3,3-dimethyl-2-(1-(pent-4-en-1-yl)-1H-indazole-3-carboxamido)butanoate—is a full and potent SCRA. It was first identified in Europe in 2017 [9], appeared in the market in mid-2019, and became one of the most common SCRA in the next year and a half [10–12]. It quickly became one of the prisons' most commonly detected SCRA [13,14]. Additionally, there are reports that cannabis is regularly adulterated with MDMB-4en-PINACA [14,15]. MDMB-4en-PINACA concentrations in these adulterated cannabis flower samples ranged from 0.3 to 4.6 µg/mg, whereas in hashish samples, it varied from 1.7 to 7.2 µg/mg [15].

MDMB-4en-PINACA shares structural features with several SCRAs, including 4F-MDMB-BINACA and 5F-MDMB-PINACA. Similarly to these compounds, MDMB-4en-PINACA contains an indazole core, a carboxamide link, and a tert-leucinate (dimethyl methyl butanoate) group. However, it differs in the tail from these compounds; it has a pent-4-ene moiety on a pentyl tail (Figure 1).

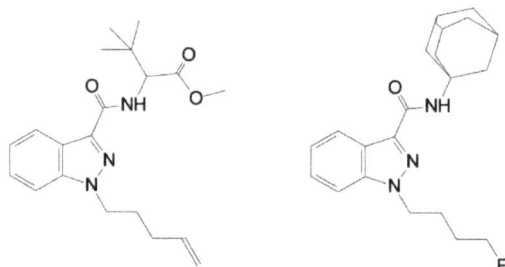

Figure 1. Chemical structure of MDMB-4en-PINACA (**left**) and 4F-ABUTINACA (**right**).

4F-ABUTINACA—also known as N-(4-fluorobutyl)-APINACA or 4F-ABINACA, with the IUPAC name N-(1-adamantyl)-1-(4-fluorobutyl)indazole-3-carboxamide—is a fourth generation indazole-adamantyl-derived SCRA (Figure 1). Its chemical structure is most similar to APINACA (AKB48) and 5F-APINACA (5F-AKB48), which are potent agonists of both the CB1 receptor and the CB2 receptor [16]. 4F-ABUTINACA appeared in Asia in 2020, but no data are available about its pharmacological properties [17–19].

Based on in vitro biological activity assessment at cannabinoid type 1 (CB1) receptor via its interaction with β-arrestin 2, the potency and efficacy of MDMB-4en-PINACA is similar to that of their structural analogs 4F-MDMB-BINACA and 5F-MDMB-PINACA. In vitro studies showed an EC50 of 1.88–2.47 nM, an Emax of 221–299% (compared to JWH-018), and a Ki value of 0.28 on the CB1 receptor [20–23]. MDMB-4en-PINACA seems to have a seven-fold greater affinity to cannabinoid type 2 (CB2) receptor than CB1 receptor [24].

Since MDMB-4en-PINACA has not been formally studied in humans, information about its pharmacological properties is limited [1]. An in vivo study revealed that MDMB-4en-PINACA interferes with hippocampal functions and impairs cognitive performance, highlighting the cognitive harm posed by MDMB-4en-PINACA [25].

It metabolizes rapidly [26], with an in vitro half-life (t1/2) of 9.1 min [1]. Gu et coworkers found that MDMB-4en-PINACA metabolism involves 11 metabolic pathways, including acetylation, a novel metabolic pathway for SCRAs. According to their findings, the major metabolic pathways involved in MDMB-4en-PINACA metabolism are ester hydrolysis and hydroxylation, and up to nine metabolites can be detected in the serum [27]. Xiang et al. also identified further ketone metabolites and special phase II metabolites [28]. Various clinical symptoms were reported after using MDMB-4en-PINACA, such as headaches, seizures, paranoia, anxiety, hallucinations, amnesia, mydriasis, nausea, and vomiting [29,30].

The European Monitoring Centre reported four deaths with confirmed exposure to MDMB-4en-PINACA for Drugs and Drug Addiction (EMCDDA). These cases occurred between 2019 and 2020, but the details were not published [31].

At the time of writing, this is the first fatal case report involving 4F-ABUTINACA reported with detailed autopsy findings and concentrations.

2. Case Report

The deceased was a 26-year-old Caucasian male with no prior medical history. He had a long history of abusing new psychoactive substances (NPS) and had previously committed multiple drug-related offenses. He was wearing an electronic tagging device at the time of his death. He had complained of acute headache and angina the day before his death. On the morning of his death, he went to the restroom at approximately 5:45 a.m. He returned to his room a few minutes later. In a short while, his father heard a thump and entered his room. The victim had a weak pulse and noisy breathing (death rattle). The father immediately called an ambulance and began resuscitation. The emergency medical personnel noticed pulseless electrical activity. Resuscitation efforts were unsuccessful, and he was pronounced dead at the scene. The police found 6.82 g of dried, shredded, green plant material in a mini zip log bag and a few cigarette butts.

Analysis of the seized green plant material and cigarette butt was carried out by the exclusively authorized national laboratory (Hungarian Institute of Forensic Sciences), MDMB-4en-PINACA and 4F-ABUTINACA were detected in each sample. The authors received the results of this analysis 24 months after the autopsy.

3. Materials and Methods

3.1. Autopsy and Sampling

Forensic autopsy was performed according to the Recommendation No.R (99)3 of the Council of Europe [32] on medico-legal autopsies. Histological samples were collected from the brain (posterior limb of the internal capsule with adjacent thalamus, rostral pons, cerebellum including the dentate nucleus, hippocampus, dorsal frontal inter-arterial watershed zone), lungs, heart (sinoatrial node, Koch's triangle (AV node), right ventricle, septum, and left ventricle), suprarenal glands, kidneys, and liver. Toxicological samples were collected from the femoral vein (whole blood) and bladder (urine).

3.2. Histology

All samples were fixed with 9% buffered formalin for three days, then stained with hematoxylin and eosin (HE). Immunohistological staining for complement factor C9 (cat. no. ABS 004-22-02, Thermo Fisher Scientific, Rockford, IL, USA) was applied on all heart samples.

3.3. Toxicological Analyses

Toxicological analyses were carried out by supercritical fluid chromatography tandem mass spectrometry (SFC-MS/MS) (Waters® ACQUITY UPC2 supercritical fluid chromatograph coupled with Xevo TQ-S triple quadrupole mass spectrometer, Milford, MA, USA), and headspace gas chromatography with flame ionization detector (HS-GC-FID) (Agilent Technologies G1888 headspace with 7890A gas chromatograph system, Santa Clara, CA, USA). Prior to the analyses, biological samples (blood and urine) were stored at 4 °C. After the analytical measurements, the samples were stored frozen (-20 °C).

SFC-MS/MS was used to identify and quantify 295 compounds, including drugs (e.g., antihypertensive drugs, anxiolytics, antipsychotics, antidepressants, antiepileptics, general and local anesthetics, NSAIDs, opioids, anticoagulants), narcotics, and novel psychoactive substances (e.g., SCRAs). In the first step of sample preparation, nine isotope-labeled internal standards were added to the samples, which cover a wide range of physicochemical properties to monitor the extraction procedure for all the target molecules. The isotope-labeled standards were amphetamine-D6, 4-methylmethcathinone-D3, delta-9-tetrahydrocannabinol-D3, 11-nor-9-carboxy-tetrahydrocannabinol-D3, N-[(1S)-1-(aminocarbonyl) -2-methylpropyl]-1-[(4-fluorophenyl)methyl]-1H-indazole-3-carboxamide D4 (AB-FUBINACA-D4), carbamazepine-D10, citalopram-D6, alprazolam-D5, and clonazepam-D4, all were purchased from Lipomed AG (Arlesheim, Switzerland). The internal standard of SCRAs was AB-FUBINACA-D4. The SCRA reference standards were obtained from the exclusively authorized national laboratory (Hungarian Institute for Forensic Sciences, Budapest, Hungary). Metabolites of SCRAs are not analyzed routinely in our laboratory.

The HS-GC-FID method was applied to determine alcohols (methanol, ethanol, 1-propanol, 2-propanol, n-butanol) and other volatiles (e.g., acetone, toluene, ethyl acetate). Tert-butanol was used as an internal standard.

The applied analytical procedures were evaluated for a number of validation characteristics (selectivity, repeatability and intermediate precision, limit of detection, limit of quantification, and calibration range).

3.3.1. SFC-MS/MS Conditions

Measurements were performed by an ACQUITY UPC2 supercritical fluid chromatography system (Waters) coupled with a Xevo TQ-S Triple Quadrupole Mass Spectrometer (Waters). Data were recorded by MassLynx software.

Separation of compounds was performed at 45 °C on a 2.1 mm × 100 mm, 1.7 μm particle size, Waters ACQUITY Torus™ DIOL analytical column with a guard cartridge (Torus™ DIOL VanGuard™, 2.1 mm × 5 mm, 130 Å, 1.7 μm). The mobile phase consisted of a mixture of carbon dioxide (A) and 10 mM ammonium hydroxide, and 12 mM formic acid in methanol/water (97.2/2.8, v/v) (B). The following gradient profile was used: 97.5% A at 0 min and 37.5% A at 10 min. A pre-equilibration period lasting 2.5 min was applied before each injection. The flow rate of the mobile phase was 0.6 mL/min, the injected volume was 0.5 μL. Constant 175 bar back pressure was used to maintain the supercritical state. To sustain a suitable electrospray, methanol was added to the mobile phase as a makeup solvent with a flow rate of 60 μL/min (Waters 515 HPLC Pump). The MS measurement was performed in positive ion mode (except for some acidic compounds such as barbiturates). The ESI source was operated with a spray voltage of 3 kV in both positive and negative ion modes. Cone voltage was 30 V. The source was set at 150 °C. Both desolvation and cone gases were nitrogen delivered at 300 and 150 L/h, respectively. Desolvation gas was tempered at 300 °C. The collision gas was argon with a flow rate of 0.13 mL/min. MS/MS experiments were performed in MRM (multiple reaction monitoring) mode with an isolation window of 0.4 m/z. MRM transitions of MDMB-4en-PINACA and 4F-ABUTINACA can be seen in Table 1.

Table 1. Analytes of interest with ionization mode, retention time (R_t), quantifier (*) and qualifier ion transitions and collision energies (CE).

Analyte	Ionization Mode	R_t (min)	Precursor Ion (m/z)	Product Ion (m/z)	CE (eV)
MDMB-4en-PINACA	ESI+	1.030	358.2	213.1 *	25
				145.0	40
				90.0	60
4F-ABUTINACA	ESI+	1.668	370.2	135.1 *	25
				107.1	45
				93.1	45

Peak detection and quantification were achieved using TargetLynx XS software (Waters). The observed ions (mass in m/z) were accepted and quantified if the following conditions were met: appropriate MS1 mass, appropriate retention time, appropriate MS2 mass, appropriate fragmentation pattern (three MRM transitions with appropriate peak area ratios), and recovery of internal standard.

3.3.2. Sample Preparation—SALLE (Salting out Assisted Liquid-Liquid Extraction)

One hundred and twenty µL of internal standard solution (125 mM formic acid/acetonitrile) was added to 90 µL of the sample. After vortex-mixing, the mixture was allowed to stand at room temperature for 5 min. In the next step, exact amount of solid ammonium formate as salting agent was added to the mixture to obtain a saturated solution at 20 °C and incubated in a thermomixer (20 °C, 1200 rpm) for 15 min. After the incubation mixture was centrifuged (18,000 rcf, 20 °C) for 5 min, 30 µL of the supernatant was transferred into a microinsert from which 0.5 µL was injected to the chromatographic system.

4. Review of the Literature

The literature was reviewed to identify reported cases of MDMB-4en-PINACA and 4F-ABUTINACA use. The search was performed on 25 July 2023 using electronic databases of PubMed, Scopus, and Web of Science (WoS) using the following search parameters: MDMB-4en-PINACA (all fields) and 4F-ABUTINACA (all fields). Conference abstracts and works in languages other than English were excluded. Results from all three databases were downloaded and collated for duplicates. Manuscripts not describing a case or cases without information on the concentration, symptoms, or autopsy findings were excluded.

5. Results

5.1. Autopsy

The autopsy was performed five days after death and documented a well-developed, athletic build man without signs of significant trauma. A puncture wound over the lateral aspect of the left cubital fossa and small abrasions on the chest were found as a result of resuscitation. Neither petechiae nor rash were identified. Internal examination revealed brain edema (1670 g), internal congestion, petechial bleeding, pleural ecchymoses, and fluidity of the blood. No anatomic cause of death was found. The results of the histopathological examination were unremarkable except for mild subendocardial fibrosis. The main macro- and microscopic findings are summarized in Table 2.

Table 2. Main autopsy and histological findings of the reported case.

Organ	Weight (g)	Macroscopical Finding	Histological Finding
Brain	1670	edema	edema
Heart	322	-[1]	minimal subendocardial fibrosis
Lung	right: 497 left: 426	congestion, edema, pleural petechial bleeding, and ecchymoses	acute congestion, minimal interstitial edema, macrophages containing double refracting brown pigments
Liver	1750	congestion	acute congestion, mild steatosis
Kidneys	302	congestion	congestion
Suprarenal gland	N/A	-[1]	congestion
Arteries	N/A	minimal atherosclerosis	-[2]

N/A: not applicable; [1] no pathological change was observed; [2] not examined.

5.2. Toxicology

Toxicological analyses determined 7.2 ng/mL of MDMB-4en-PINACA in the peripheral blood and 0.4 ng/mL in the urine. Other substances identified in the blood were caffeine (126 ng/mL) and theophylline (26 ng/mL). Ethyl alcohol could not be detected.

Blood and urine samples were re-examined 24 months after the autopsy, because analysis of the seized green plant material and cigarette butt revealed that these contained 4F-ABUTINACA in addition to MDMB-4en-PINACA. At the time of the autopsy, 4F-ABUTINACA was not routinely examined in our laboratory. The repeated toxicological analyses determined 9.1 ng/mL of 4F-ABUTINACA in the peripheral blood and 2.0 ng/mL in the urine (Figure 2). Furthermore, it turned out that MDMB-4en-PINACA is stable during long-term storage (24 months) at −20 °C both in the blood and the urine. Moreover, 103.8% of the previously determined concentration was present in unchanged form in the blood, and 100.6% in the urine. Since the stability test of 4F-ABUTINACA could not be performed, the possibility that its concentration was much higher at the time of the autopsy cannot be excluded [33].

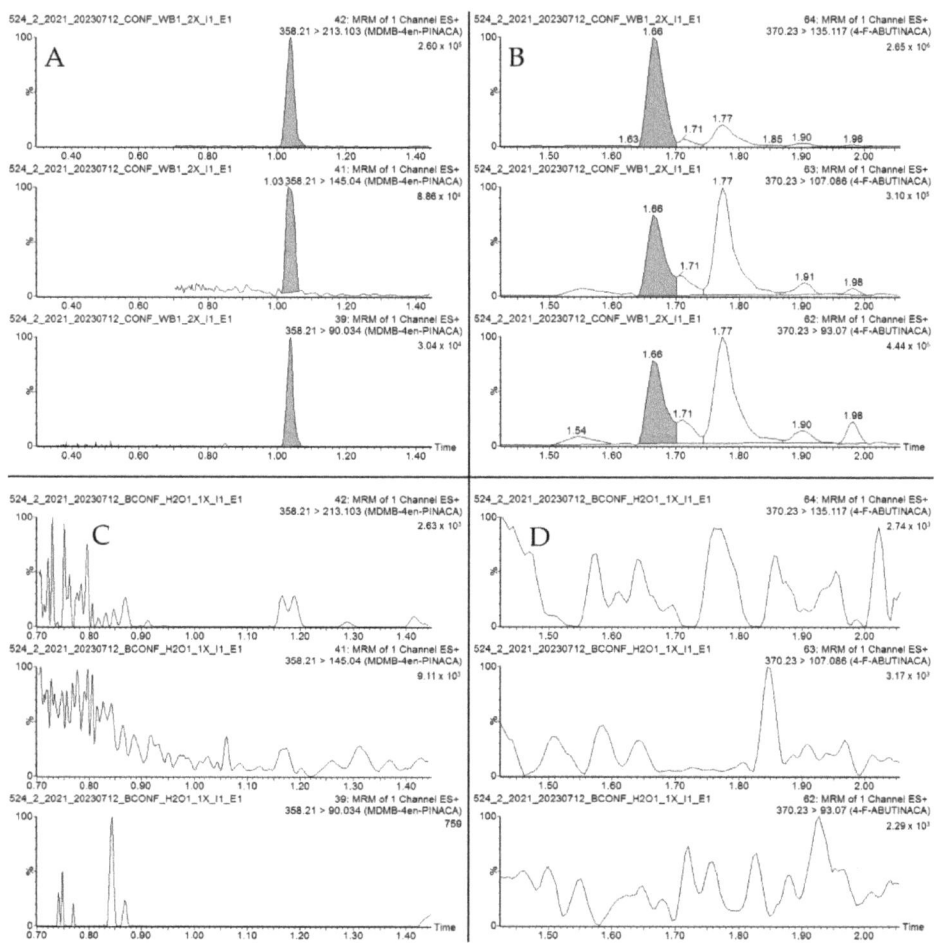

Figure 2. Representative MRM chromatograms of MDMB-4en-PINACA (**A**) and 4F-ABUTINACA (**B**) in postmortem peripheral blood sample, and corresponding chromatograms of a blank sample (**C**,**D**).

The limit of detection (LOD) of the applied method was 0.09 ng/mL for MDMB-4en-PINACA and 4F-ABUTINACA. The limit of quantification (LOQ) was 0.15 ng/mL for MDMB-4en-PINACA and 4F-ABUTINACA. Calibration range was 0.15–50.0 ng/mL for both compounds.

5.3. Review of the Literature

MDMB-4-en-PINACA was first mentioned in the scientific literature in 2019 [34]. There are now (July 2023) 44 scientific articles in all (40 entries in Pubmed, 41 in Scopus, and 37 in

Web of Science), but none of these describe a fatal case in detail, and only one describes the symptoms linked with its usage. Goncalves et al. reported eight cases of MDMB-4en-PINACA associated hospitalization with the most common symptoms of paranoia and/or hallucinations (four cases), nausea and/or vomiting (three cases), altered or loss of consciousness (three cases), psychomotor agitation and/or aggressiveness (three cases), headaches (three cases), persistent tiredness (three cases), mydriasis (three cases), seizure (two cases), amnesia (two cases), and dizziness (two cases) [29]. Seizures after consumption of MDMB-4-en-PINACA were also reported [30]. There was only one paper in which a case of a 40-year-old female was reported who died because of mixed drug toxicity, including MDMB-4-en-PINACA [35]. However, there is no information on its concentrations or any postmortem findings. Ricciardo reported a case of finding MDMB-4en-PINACA in a case of fatal thyroid storm, but they were not able to quantify the MDMB-4-en-PINACA due to prior embalming [36].

Regarding the 4F-ABUTINACA, the search revealed only one scientific article describing a UPLC method for the simultaneous determination of five indole/indazole amide-based SCRAs including 4F-ABUTINACA (article is in Chinese) [37], and it is mentioned only in one other article [38].

6. Discussion

Cardiac arrhythmias and myocardial infarction are the most common causes of death in SCRA-related fatalities, although other direct (respiratory depression, excited delirium) or indirect (accident, suicide) mechanisms are also frequent [38–41]. In fatal incidents, the most common signs and symptoms are sudden collapse, chest pain, and seizures [7]. Autopsy findings of SCRA-related fatalities are diverse. Internal congestion and edema are the most common internal findings, although other conditions, such as signs of asphyxial death, brain edema, cerebral infarction, pulmonary edema, acute respiratory distress syndrome, myocardial infarction, and acute tubular necrosis have also been observed [42,43]. Autopsy findings are unremarkable in many cases [43].

Determining the cause of death in the case of overdose of new psychoactive materials can be challenging due to the lack of data about these substances. It also presents another difficulty: the emerging new substances are often not found during the toxicological screening (so a negative screening does not exclude the possibility of an overdose). The determination of the cause of death in these cases is always based on the detection and quantification of the substances from the cadaveric blood, evaluation of the toxicological results, autopsy and histological findings (including a thorough review of the scientific literature) and excluding all other diseases or factors possibly causing the death or contributing to it. The data from scientific literature were limited in regard to the two substances detected but based on the toxicological results and after excluding other possible causes of death, the cause of death in our reported case was determined as an overdose of SCRAs, namely MDMB-4en-PINACA and 4F-ABUTINACA. However, the exact mechanism is unclear: autopsy results (brain edema, internal congestion, petechial bleeding, pleural ecchymoses, and fluidity of the blood) suggest asphyxia and, hence, respiratory depression, yet the above-described circumstances suggest a sudden collapse and potential arrhythmia. Although MDMB-4en-PINACA was one of the most commonly used SCRA in recent years, only a small number of cases have been reported, and no fatal case clearly attributed exclusively to the use of MDMB-4en-PINACA has been described in the scientific literature, and there is no manuscript describing 4F-ABUTINACA use (fatal or non-fatal).

The reported case further emphasizes that the relationship between concentration and effects in the case of SCRA use is unpredictable, with mortality occurring at relatively low concentrations, even in young and healthy individuals.

7. Conclusions

MDMB-4en-PINACA and 4F-ABUTINCA are strong, potentially lethal SCRAs; the exact effects and outcome of their use are unpredictable. MDMB-4en-PINACA and 4F-

ABUTINCA are potent, potentially lethal SCRAs; nevertheless, the precise effects and outcomes of their use are unknown.

Author Contributions: Conceptualization, G.S.; methodology, M.M. and M.K.; formal analysis, M.M. and M.K.; investigation, D.T. and K.P.; writing—original draft preparation, G.S.; writing—review and editing, D.T, M.M. and M.K.; visualization, M.K.; project administration, G.S. All authors have read and agreed to the published version of the manuscript.

Funding: This research received no external funding.

Institutional Review Board Statement: Ethical approval was waived, and the reason are already detailed below the statement section.

Informed Consent Statement: All procedures were in accordance with the 1964 Helsinki declaration and its later amendments or comparable ethical standards. Patient consent and ethical approval was waived due to it is not necessary for an anonimized case report of a forensic autopsy in the author's country. All examinations in the case report were part of the routine autopsy. The anonimized data from the autopsy can be utilized freely for scientific and educational purposes without informed consent or ethical permission according to the 40. § (3) of the Hungarian act of Forensic Experts (2016.XXIX) and 220. § (1) of the Hungarian Healthcare act of 1997.

Data Availability Statement: All data are contained within the article.

Acknowledgments: We would like to thank Tünde Wéber for her technical assistance in the toxicological analysis, and János Konrád for his help in the autopsy. We would like to thank Hungarian Institute of Forensic Sciences for SCRA reference standards.

Conflicts of Interest: The authors declare no conflict of interest.

References

1. European Monitoring Centre for Drugs and Drug Addiction. Synthetic cannabinoids in Europe—A review. 2021. Available online: https://www.emcdda.europa.eu/system/files/publications/14035/Synthetic-cannabinoids-in-Europe-EMCDDA-technical-report.pdf (accessed on 24 June 2023).
2. Bukke, V.N.; Archana, M.; Villani, R.; Serviddio, G.; Cassano, T. Pharmacological and toxicological effects of phytocannabinoids and recreational synthetic cannabinoids: Increasing risk of public health. *Pharmaceuticals* **2021**, *14*, 965. [CrossRef] [PubMed]
3. Alon, M.H.; Saint-Fleur, M.O. Synthetic cannabinoid induced acute respiratory depression: Case series and literature review. *Respir. Med. Case. Rep.* **2017**, *22*, 137–141. [CrossRef]
4. Pacher, P.; Steffens, S.; Haskó, G.; Schindler, T.H.; Kunos, G. Cardiovascular effects of marijuana and synthetic cannabinoids: The good, the bad, and the ugly. *Nat. Rev. Cardiol.* **2018**, *15*, 151–166. [CrossRef]
5. Al Fawaz, S.; Al Deeb, M.; Huffman, J.L.; Al Kholaif, N.A.; Garlich, F.; Chuang, R. A case of status epilepticus and transient stress cardiomyopathy associated with smoking the synthetic psychoactive cannabinoid, UR-144. *Am. J. Case. Rep.* **2019**, *20*, 1902–1906. [CrossRef] [PubMed]
6. Darke, S.; Banister, S.; Farrell, M.; Duflou, J.; Lappin, J. 'Synthetic cannabis': A dangerous misnomer. *Int. J. Drug. Policy* **2021**, *98*, 103396. [CrossRef] [PubMed]
7. Darke, S.; Duflou, J.; Farrell, M.; Peacock, A.; Lappin, J. Characteristics and circumstances of synthetic cannabinoid-related death. *Clin. Toxicol.* **2020**, *58*, 368–374. [CrossRef]
8. Labay, L.M.; Caruso, J.L.; Gilson, T.P.; Phipps, R.J.; Knight, L.D.; Lemos, N.P.; McIntyre, I.M.; Stoppacher, R.; Tormos, L.M.; Wiens, A.L.; et al. Synthetic cannabinoid drug use as a cause or contributory cause of death. *Forensic. Sci. Int.* **2016**, *260*, 31–39. [CrossRef] [PubMed]
9. World Health Organization. Critical Review Report: MDMB-4-en-PINACA. 2020. Available online: https://www.who.int/docs/default-source/controlled-substances/43rd-ecdd/mdmb-4en-pinaca-review-2020.pdf?sfvrsn=5cd6e97e6 (accessed on 24 June 2023).
10. Norman, C.; Walker, G.; McKirdy, B.; McDonald, C.; Fletcher, D.; Antonides, L.H.; Sutcliffe, O.B.; Nic Daéid, N.; McKenzie, C. Detection and quantitation of synthetic cannabinoid receptor agonists in infused papers from prisons in a constantly evolving illicit market. *Drug Test. Anal.* **2020**, *12*, 538–554. [CrossRef]
11. Norman, C.; Halter, S.; Haschimi, B.; Acreman, D.; Smith, J.; Krotulski, A.J.; Mohr, A.L.A.; Logan, B.K.; NicDaéid, N.; Auwärter, V.; et al. A transnational perspective on the evolution of the synthetic cannabinoid receptor agonists market: Comparing prison and general populations. *Drug Test. Anal.* **2021**, *13*, 841–852. [CrossRef]
12. Rodrigues, T.B.; Souza, M.P.; de Melo Barbosa, L.; de Carvalho Ponce, J.; Júnior, L.F.N.; Yonamine, M.; Costa, J.L. Synthetic cannabinoid receptor agonists profile in infused papers seized in Brazilian prisons. *Forensic. Toxicol.* **2022**, *40*, 119–124. [CrossRef]

13. Vaccaro, G.; Massariol, A.; Guirguis, A.; Kirton, S.B.; Stair, J.L. NPS detection in prison: A systematic literature review of use, drug form, and analytical approaches. *Drug. Test. Anal.* **2022**, *14*, 1350–1367. [CrossRef] [PubMed]
14. Oomen, P.E.; Schori, D.; Tögel-Lins, K.; Acreman, D.; Chenorhokian, S.; Luf, A.; Karden, A.; Paulos, C.; Fornero, E.; Gerace, E.; et al. Cannabis adulterated with the synthetic cannabinoid receptor agonist MDMB-4en-PINACA and the role of European drug checking services. *Int. J. Drug. Policy* **2022**, *100*, 103493. [CrossRef] [PubMed]
15. Monti, M.C.; Zeugin, J.; Koch, K.; Milenkovic, N.; Scheurer, E.; Mercer-Chalmers-Bender, K. Adulteration of low-delta-9-tetrahydrocannabinol products with synthetic cannabinoids: Results from drug checking services. *Drug. Test. Anal.* **2022**, *14*, 1026–1039. [CrossRef] [PubMed]
16. Canazza, I.; Ossato, A.; Trapella, C.; Fantinati, A.; De Luca, M.A.; Margiani, G.; Vincenzi, F.; Rimondo, C.; Di Rosa, F.; Gregori, A.; et al. Effect of the novel synthetic cannabinoids AKB48 and 5F-AKB48 on "tetrad", sensorimotor, neurological and neurochemical responses in mice. In vitro and in vivo pharmacological studies. *Psychopharmacology* **2016**, *233*, 3685–3709. [CrossRef]
17. United Nations Office on Drugs and Crime. Synthetic Drugs in East and Southeast Asia. Latest developments and Challenges. 2021. Available online: https://www.unodc.org/documents/scientific/ATS/2021_ESEA_Regional_Synthetic_Drugs_Report.pdf (accessed on 24 June 2023).
18. de Oliveira, M.C.; Vides, M.C.; Lassi, D.L.S.; Torales, J.; Ventriglio, A.; Bombana, H.S.; Leyton, V.; Périco, C.d.A.-M.; Negrão, A.B.; Malbergier, A.; et al. Toxicity of Synthetic Cannabinoids in K2/Spice: A Systematic Review. *Brain Sci.* **2023**, *13*, 990. [CrossRef]
19. Malaca, S.; Busardò, F.P.; Nittari, G.; Sirignano, A.; Ricci, G. Fourth Generation of Synthetic Cannabinoid Receptor Agonists: A Review on the Latest Insights. *Curr. Pharm. Des.* **2022**, *28*, 2603–2617. [CrossRef]
20. Krotulski, A.J.; Cannaert, A.; Stove, C.; Logan, B.K. The next generation of synthetic cannabinoids: Detection, activity, and potential toxicity of pent-4en and but-3en analogues including MDMB-4en-PINACA. *Drug Test. Anal.* **2021**, *13*, 427–438. [CrossRef]
21. Pike, E.; Grafinger, K.E.; Cannaert, A.; Ametovski, A.; Luo, J.L.; Sparkes, E.; Cairns, E.A.; Ellison, R.; Gerona, R.; Stove, C.P.; et al. Systematic evaluation of a panel of 30 synthetic cannabinoid receptor agonists structurally related to MMB-4en-PICA, MDMB-4en-PINACA, ADB-4en-PINACA, and MMB-4CN-BUTINACA using a combination of binding and different CB1 receptor activation assays: Part I-Synthesis, analytical characterization, and binding affinity for human CB1 receptors. *Drug. Test. Anal.* **2021**, *13*, 1383–1401. [CrossRef]
22. Grafinger, K.E.; Cannaert, A.; Ametovski, A.; Sparkes, E.; Cairns, E.; Banister, S.D.; Auwärter, V.; Stove, C.P. Systematic evaluation of a panel of 30 synthetic cannabinoid receptor agonists structurally related to MMB-4en-PICA, MDMB-4en-PINACA, ADB-4en-PINACA, and MMB-4CN-BUTINACA using a combination of binding and different CB1 receptor activation assays-Part II: Structure activity relationship assessment via a β-arrestin recruitment assay. *Drug Test. Anal.* **2021**, *13*, 1402–1411. [CrossRef]
23. Cannaert, A.; Sparkes, E.; Pike, E.; Luo, J.L.; Fang, A.; Kevin, R.C.; Ellison, R.; Gerona, R.; Banister, S.D.; Stove, C.P. Synthesis and in vitro cannabinoid receptor 1 activity of recently detected synthetic cannabinoids 4F-MDMB-BICA, 5F-MPP-PICA, MMB-4en-PICA, CUMYL-CBMICA, ADB-BINACA, APP-BINACA, 4F-MDMB-BINACA, MDMB-4en-PINACA, A-CHMINACA, 5F-AB-P7AICA, 5F-MDMB-P7AICA, and 5F-AP7AICA. *ACS. Chem. Neurosci.* **2020**, *11*, 4434–4446. [CrossRef]
24. Marusich, J.A.; Gamage, T.F.; Zhang, Y.; Akinfiresoye, L.R.; Wiley, J.L. In vitro and in vivo pharmacology of nine novel synthetic cannabinoid receptor agonists. *Pharmacol. Biochem. Behav.* **2022**, *220*, 173467. [CrossRef] [PubMed]
25. Ali, S.M.; Kolieb, E.; Imbaby, S.; Hagras, A.M.; Korayem Arafat, H.E.; Kamel, E.M.; Abdelshakour, M.A.; Mohammed Ali, M.I. Acute toxic effects of new synthetic cannabinoid on brain: Neurobehavioral and Histological: Preclinical studies. *Chem. Biol. Interact.* **2023**, *370*, 110306. [CrossRef] [PubMed]
26. Erol Ozturk, Y.; Yeter, O. In vitro phase I metabolism of the recently emerged synthetic MDMB-4en-PINACA and its detection in human urine samples. *J. Anal. Toxicol.* **2021**, *44*, 976–984. [CrossRef] [PubMed]
27. Gu, K.; Qin, S.; Zhang, Y.; Zhang, W.; Xin, G.; Shi, B.; Wang, J.; Wang, Y.; Lu, J. Metabolic profiles and screening tactics for MDMB-4en-PINACA in human urine and serum samples. *J. Pharm. Biomed. Anal.* **2022**, *220*, 114985. [CrossRef]
28. Xiang, J.; Wen, D.; Zhao, J.; Xiang, P.; Shi, Y.; Ma, C. Study of the Metabolic Profiles of "Indazole-3-Carboxamide" and "Isatin Acyl Hydrazone" (OXIZID) Synthetic Cannabinoids in a Human Liver Microsome Model Using UHPLC-QE Orbitrap MS. *Metabolites* **2023**, *13*, 576. [CrossRef]
29. Goncalves, R.; Labadie, M.; Chouraqui, S.; Peyré, A.; Castaing, N.; Daveluy, A.; Molimard, M. Involuntary MDMB-4en-PINACA intoxications following cannabis consumption: Clinical and analytical findings. *Clin. Toxicol.* **2022**, *60*, 458–463. [CrossRef]
30. Goncalves, R.; Peyré, A.; Castaing, N.; Beeken, T.; Olivier, S.; Combe, P.; Miremont-Salamé, G.; Titier, K.; Molimard, M.; Daveluy, A. Minors and young adult's hospitalizations after "chimique" consumption in Mayotte Island: Which substances are involved? *Therapie* **2023**, *78*, 235–240. [CrossRef]
31. EMCDDA Initial Report on the New Psychoactive Substance Methyl 3,3-Dimethyl-2-(1-(pent-4-en-1-yl)-1H-indazole-3-carboxamido)butanoate (MDMB-4en-PINACA). 2020. Available online: https://www.emcdda.europa.eu/publications/initial-reports/mdmb-4en-pinaca_en (accessed on 24 June 2023).
32. Council of Europe Comitee of Ministers. Recommendation No.R (99)3 on the Harmonization of Medico-legal Autopsy Rules. 1999. Available online: https://www.coe.int/t/dg3/healthbioethic/texts_and_documents/RecR(99)3.pdf (accessed on 24 June 2023).

33. Szpot, P.; Nowak, K.; Wachełko, O.; Tusiewicz, K.; Chłopaś-Konowałek, A.; Zawadzki, M. Methyl (S)-2-(1–7 (5-fluoropentyl)-1H-indole-3-carboxamido)-3,3-dimethylbutanoate (5F-MDMB-PICA) intoxication in a child with identification of two new metabolites (ultra-high-performance liquid chromatography–tandem mass spectrometry). *Forensic Toxicol.* **2023**, *41*, 47–58. [CrossRef] [PubMed]
34. Watanabe, S.; Vikingsson, S.; Åstrand, A.; Gréen, H.; Kronstrand, R. Biotransformation of the new synthetic cannabinoid with an alkene, MDMB-4en-PINACA, by human hepatocytes, human liver microsomes, and human urine and blood. *AAPS J.* **2019**, *22*, 13. [CrossRef]
35. Rice, K.; Hikin, L.; Lawson, A.; Smith, P.R.; Morley, S. Quantification of flualprazolam in blood by LC–MS-MS: A case series of nine deaths. *J. Anal. Toxicol.* **2021**, *45*, 410–416. [CrossRef]
36. Ricciardo, S.; Hastings, S. Fatal Thyroid Storm in the Setting of Untreated Graves Disease and Use of the Synthetic Cannabinoid MDMB-4en-PINACA. *Am. J. Forensic Med. Pathol.* **2023**. [CrossRef] [PubMed]
37. Yang, Z.; Lyu, J.X.; Wu, Y.D.; Jiang, L.W.; Li, D.M. Simultaneous determination of five indole/indazole amide-based synthetic cannabinoids in electronic cigarette oil by ultra performance liquid chromatography. *Chin. J. Chromatogr.* **2023**, *41*, 602–609. [CrossRef] [PubMed]
38. Hancox, J.C.; Kalk, N.J.; Henderson, G. Synthetic cannabinoids and potential cardiac arrhythmia risk: An important message for drug users. *Ther. Adv. Drug. Saf.* **2020**, *11*, 2042098620913416. [CrossRef] [PubMed]
39. Giorgetti, A.; Busardò, F.P.; Tittarelli, R.; Auwärter, V.; Giorgetti, R. Post-mortem toxicology: A systematic review of death cases involving synthetic cannabinoid receptor agonists. *Front. Psychiatry* **2020**, *11*, 464. [CrossRef]
40. Simon, G.; Tóth, D.; Heckmann, V.; Mayer, M.; Kuzma, M. Simultaneous fatal poisoning of two victims with 4F-MDMB-BINACA and ethanol. *Forensic Toxicol.* **2023**, *41*, 151–157. [CrossRef]
41. Simon, G.; Tóth, D.; Heckmann, V.; Kuzma, M.; Mayer, M. Lethal case of myocardial ischemia following overdose of the synthetic cannabinoid ADB-FUBINACA. *Leg. Med.* **2022**, *54*, 102004. [CrossRef]
42. Logan, B.K.; Mohr, A.L.A.; Friscia, M.; Krotulski, A.J.; Papsun, D.M.; Kacinko, S.L.; Ropero-Miller, J.D.; Huestis, M.A. Reports of adverse events associated with use of novel psychoactive substances, 2013–2016, A review. *J. Anal. Toxicol.* **2017**, *41*, 573–610. [CrossRef]
43. Mohr, A.L.A.; Logan, B.K.; Fogarty, M.F.; Krotulski, A.J.; Papsun, D.M.; Kacinko, S.L.; Huestis, M.A.; Ropero-Miller, J.D. Reports of adverse events associated with use of novel psychoactive substances, 2017–2020, A review. *J. Anal. Toxicol.* **2022**, *46*, e116–e185. [CrossRef]

Disclaimer/Publisher's Note: The statements, opinions and data contained in all publications are solely those of the individual author(s) and contributor(s) and not of MDPI and/or the editor(s). MDPI and/or the editor(s) disclaim responsibility for any injury to people or property resulting from any ideas, methods, instructions or products referred to in the content.

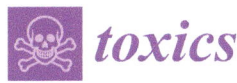

Case Report

Biodetoxification Using Intravenous Lipid Emulsion, a Rescue Therapy in Life-Threatening Quetiapine and Venlafaxine Poisoning: A Case Report

Cristian Cobilinschi [1,2], Liliana Mirea [1,2,*], Cosmin-Andrei Andrei [1,2,*], Raluca Ungureanu [1,2], Ana-Maria Cotae [1,2], Oana Avram [3,4], Sebastian Isac [5,6], Ioana Marina Grințescu [1,2] and Radu Țincu [3,4]

1. Department of Anesthesiology and Intensive Care II, Carol Davila University of Medicine, and Pharmacy, 050474 Bucharest, Romania; cristian.cobilinschi@umfcd.ro (C.C.)
2. Department of Anesthesiology and Intensive Care, Clinical Emergency Hospital Bucharest, 014461 Bucharest, Romania
3. Department of Clinical Toxicology, Carol Davila University of Medicine, and Pharmacy, 050474 Bucharest, Romania; r_tincu@yahoo.com (R.Ț.)
4. Department of Anesthesiology and Intensive Care Toxicology, Clinical Emergency Hospital Bucharest, 014461 Bucharest, Romania
5. Department of Physiology, Carol Davila University of Medicine, and Pharmacy, 050474 Bucharest, Romania
6. Department of Anesthesiology and Intensive Care, Fundeni Clinical Institute, 022328 Bucharest, Romania
* Correspondence: llmirea@yahoo.com (L.M.); andreicosmin1994@gmail.com (C.-A.A.)

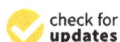

Citation: Cobilinschi, C.; Mirea, L.; Andrei, C.-A.; Ungureanu, R.; Cotae, A.-M.; Avram, O.; Isac, S.; Grințescu, I.M.; Țincu, R. Biodetoxification Using Intravenous Lipid Emulsion, a Rescue Therapy in Life-Threatening Quetiapine and Venlafaxine Poisoning: A Case Report. *Toxics* **2023**, *11*, 917. https://doi.org/10.3390/toxics11110917

Academic Editor: Eric J. F. Franssen

Received: 3 October 2023
Revised: 30 October 2023
Accepted: 7 November 2023
Published: 9 November 2023

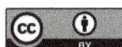

Copyright: © 2023 by the authors. Licensee MDPI, Basel, Switzerland. This article is an open access article distributed under the terms and conditions of the Creative Commons Attribution (CC BY) license (https://creativecommons.org/licenses/by/4.0/).

Abstract: The administration of intravenous lipid emulsion (ILE) is a proven antidote used to reverse local anesthetic-related systemic toxicity. Although the capacity of ILE to generate blood tissue partitioning of lipophilic drugs has been previously demonstrated, a clear recommendation for its use as an antidote for other lipophilic drugs is still under debate. Venlafaxine (an antidepressant acting as a serotonin–norepinephrine reuptake inhibitor (SNRI)) and quetiapine (a second-generation atypical antipsychotic) are widely used in the treatment of psychotic disorders. Both are lipophilic drugs known to induce cardiotoxicity and central nervous depression. We report the case of a 33-year-old man with a medical history of schizoaffective disorder who was admitted to the emergency department (ED) after having been found unconscious due to a voluntary ingestion of 12 g of quetiapine and 4.5 g of venlafaxine. Initial assessment revealed a cardiorespiratory stable patient but unresponsive with a GCS of 4 (M2 E1 V1). In the ED, he was intubated, and gastric lavage was performed. Immediately after the admission to the intensive care unit (ICU), his condition quickly deteriorated, developing cardiovascular collapse refractory to crystalloids and vasopressor infusion. Junctional bradycardia occurred, followed by spontaneous conversion to sinus rhythm. Subsequently, frequent ventricular extrasystoles, as well as patterns of bigeminy, trigeminy, and even episodes of non-sustained ventricular tachycardia, occurred. Additionally, generalized tonic–clonic seizures were observed. Alongside supportive therapy, antiarrhythmic and anticonvulsant therapy, intravenous lipid emulsion bolus, and continuous infusion were administered. His condition progressively improved over the following hours, and 24 h later, he was tapered off the vasopressor. On day 2, the patient repeated the cardiovascular collapse and a second dose of ILE was administered. Over the next few days, the patient's clinical condition improved, and he was successfully weaned off ventilator and vasopressor support. ILE has the potential to become a form of rescue therapy in cases of severe lipophilic drug poisoning and should be considered a viable treatment for severe cardiovascular instability that is refractory to supportive therapy.

Keywords: intravenous lipid emulsion; antidote; venlafaxine; quetiapine; suicidal attempt; cardiotoxicity; neurotoxicity; intoxication

1. Introduction

Suicide by drug overdose can be precipitated by a variety of factors, such as psychiatric disorders like depression, anxiety, bipolar disorder, and schizophrenia, among others. Typically, venlafaxine and quetiapine are prescribed to treat these types of disorders.

Quetiapine is an antipsychotic drug belonging to the class of dibenzothiazepine. Low to moderate antagonist activity at multiple neurotransmitter receptor sites is described, such as serotonergic 5-hydroxytryptamine (5-HT2A) receptors, dopaminergic (D1 and D2) receptors, histaminergic (H1) receptors, adrenergic $\alpha1$ and $\alpha2$ receptors, and partial agonist activity at 5-HT1A receptors [1]. In a 5-year retrospective analysis of 945 cases diagnosed with acute quetiapine overdose, the main clinical manifestations were drowsiness (76%), coma (10%), seizures (2%), tachycardia (56%), hypotension (18%), and respiratory depression (5%), complications that were more commonly compared with overdose of all other antipsychotic agents [2].

Venlafaxine is a phenethylamine derivative, a selective serotonin and norepinephrine reuptake inhibitor (SNRI). It acts by raising neurotransmitter levels in the brain, which can enhance mood and alleviate symptoms of depression and anxiety [3]. Venlafaxine has been reported to be notably more toxic than selective serotonin reuptake inhibitors (SSRIs) [4]. Clinical manifestations of an overdose of venlafaxine include nausea, vomiting, seizures, agitation, confusion, and changes in blood pressure or heart rate. In critical cases, the overdose may lead to coma, acute respiratory failure, or cardiac arrest. It is also associated with a high prevalence of cardiovascular adverse events. When cardiotoxicity arises, it can manifest itself in a serious manner, as seen in cases of Takotsubo cardiomyopathy, acute coronary syndromes with normal coronary arteries, and malignant arrhythmias. A recent investigation showed that severe cardiotoxicity occurs if the ingestion dose is greater than 8 g, but this is not paramount. Tachycardia and QTc interval prolongation appears to be a dose-dependent effect that may lead to severe cardiac arrhythmias [5–7]. If the ingestion dose exceeds 8 g, patients could also manifest other symptoms, including seizures and serotonin toxicity.

The two drugs are often used to treat mental health conditions. Quetiapine is used to treat schizophrenia, bipolar disorder, and major depressive disorder, whereas venlafaxine is used to treat depression and anxiety disorders. An overdose of either of these drugs can be fatal and necessitates emergency medical intervention. The particular symptoms of an overdose may differ depending on the amount of medication used, as well as individual patient characteristics, such as age and overall health.

Intravenous lipid emulsion (ILE) therapy was initially proposed to address systemic toxicity caused by local anesthetics [8]. Recent case reports have indicated that lipid emulsion infusion may be an effective treatment for non-local anesthetic overdoses involving a diverse range of drugs, including beta-blockers, calcium channel blockers, parasiticides, herbicides, and several psychiatric substances. ILE has been used to treat severe toxicity caused by a variety of lipophilic drugs [9,10]. Even low doses of intravenous lipid emulsion infusion have been reported to be a possibly useful therapy in quetiapine overdose [11]. There are currently no dosage guidelines for drug toxicity other than local anesthetics.

In this study, we report a case involving a deliberate overdose of quetiapine and venlafaxine, which resulted in a life-threatening situation. However, the patient in question was successfully treated using intravenous lipid emulsion (ILE) therapy.

2. Case Report

We report the case of a 33-year-old man with a medical history of schizoaffective disorder, who was admitted to the emergency department (ED) after having been found unconscious due to a voluntary ingestion of 12 g of quetiapine and 4.5 g of venlafaxine. Ingestion was estimated to occur 8 h before presentation. Upon initial assessment, the patient was spontaneous breathing; he was normotensive but comatose with a Glasgow Coma Scale of 4 points (M2 E1 V1) with midline symmetrical dilated pupils and preserved light responses. Considering the patient's neurological state, he was intubated, and mechanical ventilation was initiated. Gastrointestinal decontamination was promptly performed, consisting of gastric lavage and administration of activated charcoal.

Initial laboratory tests were within normal limits, although the first arterial blood gas analysis revealed elevated lactate of 5.3 m Mol/L. Urine was analyzed by qualitative gas chromatography–mass spectrometry, which was positive for venlafaxine and quetiapine. Additionally, 12 leads electrocardiography (ECG) was recorded without revealing significant changes. The initial QTc interval was assessed at 456 ms.

The patient was admitted to the toxicology intensive care unit, where his condition rapidly deteriorated, developing cardiovascular collapse. The patient's systolic blood pressure had a downward trend despite volume resuscitation with balanced crystalloids and synthetic colloids. Additionally, vasopressor therapy was initiated with a norepinephrine infusion in doses up to 0.4 µg/kg/min. However, the cardiovascular collapse exhibited resistance to vasopressor intervention and volume resuscitation, resulting in an ongoing decline in blood pressure. Subsequently, the occurrence of junctional bradycardia was observed, which was followed by the spontaneous restoration to sinus rhythm. Subsequently, frequent ventricular extrasystoles, as well as patterns of bigeminy, trigeminy, and even episodes of nonsustained ventricular tachycardia, occurred. In addition, the patient also exhibited generalized tonic–clonic seizures.

A repeated ECG revealed a prolonged QTc of 510 ms. A transthoracic echocardiography exam showed a hyperdynamic left ventricle without abnormalities in wall motion. No right ventricle (RV) dysfunction was registered.

Alongside supportive therapy, antiarrhythmic and anticonvulsant therapy were initiated. Due to severe cardiotoxicity, lipid emulsion 20% (Intralipid® 20%, Fresenius Kabi, Bucharest, Romania) was administered as an intravenous bolus: 1.5 mL/kg over 1 min~100 mL. This was followed by a 0.1 mL/kg/min (approximately 400 mL/h) 2 h continuous infusion. Intravenous magnesium sulphate was administered 18 h post-ingestion when the QTc was 510 ms. The patient's condition progressively improved over the following hours, and he was weaned off the vasopressor within 90 min of ILE therapy initiation (Table 1).

Table 1. Timeframe in hours following ingestion and clinical and paraclinical markers.

Timeframe (hours following ingestion)	0	12	14	16	18	20	22	24	48	55	72	96	120
Lactate (mmol/L)		5.3	4.3	3.6	4.7	3.5	3.3	3.1	2.2	3.6	2.0	1.5	1
Noradrenaline (mcg/kg/min)				0.25	0.4	0.14	0	0	0	0.2	0.13	0	0
QTc (ms)		456		510				503			480		440
ILE therapy					*					**			

* Intralipid 20%® 1.5 mL/kg—100 mL intravenous bolus over 1 min, followed by a 0.1 mL/kg/min 2-h continuous infusion. ** Intralipid 20%® 1.5 mL/kg—100 mL intravenous bolus over 1 min.

On the second ICU day (55 h after ingestion), the patient became hypotensive, requiring vasopressor therapy with noradrenaline in a dose of ~0.2 µg/kg/min. This was followed by sinus bradycardia, which was managed with the help of an atropine bolus. Additionally, a second dose of ILE 1.5 mL/kg was administered.

Over the course of the patient's stay in the ICU, multiple ECGs were recorded, revealing normalization of QTc after day 6 of ICU. In addition, until day 6 of the patient's stay in ICU, the urine toxicological exam remained positive for both quetiapine and venlafaxine.

Hypertriglyceridemia, pancreatitis, and phlebitis, which are common side effects of ILE therapy, were not observed in this case.

Over the next few days, the patient's clinical condition improved. Sedation was successfully stopped, and afterwards, the patient was weaned from vasopressors and successfully extubated. One week after ingestion, he returned to his neurological baseline. On day 15, the patient was discharged in good clinical condition and referred to a psychiatrist specialist to manage the suicidal attempt.

3. Discussion

There is currently no known specific treatment for quetiapine and venlafaxine overdose. In instances where there are more severe symptoms, it is advisable to admit the patient to an intensive care unit where supportive care will be used, such as assuring proper airway, oxygenation, and ventilation, monitoring heart rate and vital signs indicators. Additionally, symptomatic measures are advised. It is not recommended to induce emesis. If performed promptly after intake, gastric lavage may be indicated. Activated charcoal should be used. Due to the large volume of distribution of these drugs, forced diuresis, dialysis, hemoperfusion, and exchange transfusion are unlikely to be of benefit. There are no particular antidotes for venlafaxine or quetiapine overdoses. Intravenous lipid emulsion (ILE) infusion has been reported to be a possibly useful therapy when other interventions have failed [11,12]. Extracorporeal life support should be employed in severe cases of drug-induced cardiotoxicity [13].

Antidepressant poisoning most commonly manifests similarly to serotonin syndrome symptoms, such as high fever, convulsions, mydriasis, and unconsciousness; however, overdose may also cause cardiotoxicity by inhibiting various cardiac ion channels, resulting in sinus bradycardia and QT or QRS prolongation [14]. Atypical antipsychotic overdoses are associated with significantly higher mortality rates. Antipsychotic-induced cardiotoxicity is also caused by alpha-1-adrenergic antagonism, which causes vasoplegia and reflex tachycardia due to antimuscarinic action [15].

The management of patients who have overdosed on both venlafaxine and quetiapine is determined by the degree of overdose and the symptoms that the patient is experiencing. Overdoses of these medications can be fatal.

The immediate release of quetiapine has a linear pharmacokinetic profile with an elimination half-life ($t_{\frac{1}{2}}$) of approximately 6–7 h, reaching a peak plasma concentration at 1–1.5 h after ingestion. Additionally, immediate release from the elimination of venlafaxine $t_{\frac{1}{2}}$ is 5 ± 2 h. Extended release from the elimination of $t_{\frac{1}{2}}$ is 15 ± 6 h. Because plasma concentrations of quetiapine and venlafaxine in this patient were not measured, it is unclear whether the patient's clearance or metabolism of these drugs was abnormal. Therefore, the second peak of toxicity occurred at 55 h, and it is not clear if it was related to the extended released form of these drugs. This could have been something associated with the late occurrence of cardiotoxicity.

The utilization of ILE therapy has been well recognized as an effective approach to managing local anesthetics systemic toxicity (LAST). Professional bodies such as the American Society of Regional Anesthesia (ASRA) endorse the use of intravenous lipid emulsion (ILE) therapy, referred to as lipid resuscitation therapy (LRT), as the recommended treatment for LAST [16]. Starting with the 2015 American Heart Association guidelines for "Special Circumstances of Resuscitation", the use of ILE therapy is recommended as a supplementary approach to advanced cardiac life support techniques in cases of suspected cardiac arrest produced by local anesthetic systemic toxicity (LAST) [17].

Additionally, ILE therapy has been employed to treat severe toxicity caused by a variety of lipophilic drugs [9,10]. The mechanism through which lipophilic drug toxicity is treated using ILE therapy is most likely a complex one [12,18]. "The lipid sink theory" hypothesizes that a lipid emulsion traps the drug in the intravascular compartment, preventing it from reaching the peripheral tissues and organs. The reduction in toxicity is achieved by decreasing the concentration of the toxin at the site of its effect. In addition to scavenging, both animal and human models have demonstrated the existence of cardiotonic and postconditioning effects resulting from lipid infusion. Lipids have a direct impact on enhancing cardiac contractility, leading to an improvement in cardiac output and an increase in preload via direct volume expansion [19,20]. However, a growing body of evidence supports the contribution of other mechanisms, such as providing cardiomyocytes with enough free fatty acids used as an alternate energy source and generating a direct positive inotropic effect. Other mechanisms include calcium and sodium channel modulation and vasoplegia reduction via endothelial nitric oxide synthase inhibition [21–23].

In 2016, the literature was analyzed by a collaborative workgroup, which subsequently formulated clinical guidance regarding the utilization of intravenous lipid emulsion in cases of drug overdose limited only to a few specific situations [24]. Numerous practical aspects, such as the optimal dose, the optimal administration time frame, and the optimal duration of infusion for clinical efficacy, as well as the threshold dose for adverse effects, are still being debated. Current knowledge substantiates the utilization of ILE exclusively in cases of LAST and cardiac toxicity caused by lipophilic drugs when an imminent risk to the patient's life and alternative treatments have proved to be inefficacious. The use of ILE as a potential antidote is still in its early stages, and more preclinical investigations, clinical studies, and systematic reporting of its usage in humans are required before any recommendations can be made. There is limited comprehension regarding ILE effectiveness, its mechanism of action, and safety [25].

The primary source of information regarding side effects pertains to the administration of intravenous lipids as a form of parenteral nutrition. These adverse effects encompass allergic reactions, hypertriglyceridemia, pancreatitis, bacteremia, fat embolism, thrombophlebitis with peripheral administration, heart failure, lipoid pneumonia, and acute respiratory distress syndrome (ARDS) [26].

Toxicology experts currently recommend a 1.5 mL/kg lean body mass of 20% lipid emulsion bolus followed by a continuous infusion of 0.25 mL/kg/min, with options to repeat the bolus or double the infusion rate for persistent cardiovascular instability [27].

The initial documentation of the successful use of lipid emulsion as an antidote for lipophilic, non-local anesthetic toxicity in a human subject was reported in a case involving a 17-year-old female who ingested a substantial amount of bupropion and lamotrigine, resulting in a severe cardiovascular collapse unresponsive to standard advanced cardiovascular life support. A 20% intravenous lipid emulsion was administered as a rescue intervention in an effort to restore hemodynamics, leading to the normalization of vital signs within one minute [28].

In a case series report, intravenous lipid emulsion was administered for the treatment of various lipophilic drug intoxications, resulting in the amelioration of cardiovascular and neurologic symptoms. The report concluded that ILE treatment is an effective lifesaving intervention for lipophilic drug intoxications, particularly in unconscious patients presenting with cardiac and/or neurologic manifestations [9].

A case report of a 34-year-old patient with a mixed overdose of multiple lipid-soluble drugs documented effects such as a notable decrease in the degree of consciousness and a severe circulatory collapse that did not respond to treatment with adrenaline, noradrenaline, and vasopressin. Additionally, the patient had significant acidemia. However, the clinical condition of the patient began to improve after receiving a lipid infusion, which resulted in a quick reduction in the need for inotropic and vasopressor support, as well as the correction of acidosis [29].

A previous case report also details the effective utilization of ILE therapy for a 61-year-old male patient who purposefully ingested excessive quantities of quetiapine and sertraline. Upon arrival at the emergency department, the patient was assessed with a score of 3, according to the Glasgow Coma Scale, and was hypotensive. Around four hours after consumption, a bolus dose of 1.5 mL/kg of a 20% lipid emulsion was administered, followed by an infusion of 6 mL/kg (400 mL). Within fifteen minutes, a notable improvement in the patient's level of consciousness was registered, resulting in a Glasgow Coma Scale (GCS) score of 9 [30].

Another case report describes a patient with acute quetiapine overdose, leading to circulatory collapse. Attempts to stabilize the patient's condition with vasopressor/inotropic therapy were ineffective. However, the administration of intravenous lipid emulsion (ILE) successfully restored cardiovascular stability [31].

Table 2 contains data from multiple case reports when intravenous lipid therapy was successfully used for acute intoxication with drugs that included quetiapine and/or venlafaxine. Each case described in the table includes the dosing and timing of ILE therapy and the symptoms for which intravenous lipid therapy was used.

Table 2. Case reports on acute intoxications that included quetiapine and/or venlafaxine, in which intravenous lipid emulsion therapy was used.

Reference	Drug	Symptoms	ILE Dose	Timing ILE Therapy	Clinical Outcome
Finn et al. [30]	Quetiapine and sertraline	GCS 3 points	20% lipid emulsion IV bolus dose of 1.5 mL/kg (100 mL) followed by an infusion of 6 mL/kg (400 mL)	4 h after ingestion	Rapid and sustained rise in consciousness (GCS 9) occurred simultaneously with ILE therapy
Bartos and Knudsen [31]	Quetiapine	Cardiovascular collapse refractory to vasopressor treatment and volume resuscitation	20% lipid emulsion IV bolus dose of 170 mL followed by an infusion of 500 mL 20% lipid emulsion run over 1 h		Within the first hour, vasopressor requirement decreased and no further boluses of either epinephrine or phenylephrine were required
Engin et al. [32]	Quetiapine	Depressed consciousness, tachycardia, and hypotension	Two 1.5-mL/kg 20% lipid emulsion IV bolus doses 15 min apart with no infusion drip	One hour after admission to the ICU, ILE therapy was considered to prevent further complications	Symptoms improved
Cevik et al. [9]	Quetiapine	Hypotension and sinus tachycardia	100 mL 20% lipid emulsion IV bolus, followed by 30 mL kg/h infusion over 2 h (total dose of 3580 mL)		Hypotension and tachycardia regressed two hours after ILE treatment
Hieger et al. [33]	Quetiapine	Status epilepticus and cardiovascular collapse	1.5-mL/kg 20% lipid emulsion IV bolus over 5 min, then a drip at 0.25 mL/kg/min (total dose 2000 mL)	11 h after ingestion	Norepinephrine was discontinued
Harvey et al. [34]	Mixed overdose, including Quetiapine and Amitriptyline	Hemodynamic instability with prolonged QRS and QTc	100 mL 20% lipid emulsion IV bolus over 1 min followed by a further 400 mL over 30 min		Hemodynamics improved, QRS and QTc normalized
Purg et al. [11]	Quetiapine, Citalopram, Bromazepam	Life-threatening arrhythmia (prolonged QTc followed by PVC and VT with pules) and status epilepticus	1.5 mL/kg (100 mL) 20% lipid emulsion IV bolus over 10 min, followed by an additional 200 mL over the next hours	12 h after admission	After ILE, QTc normalized, and ventricular tachycardia and seizures stopped

Table 2. Cont.

Reference	Drug	Symptoms	ILE Dose	Timing ILE Therapy	Clinical Outcome
De Wit et al. [35]	Venlafaxine	MODS and refractory shock	1.5 mL/kg (120 mL) 20% lipid emulsion IV as a single bolus dose	40 h after presumed ingestion	Following the administration of the intravenous lipid emulsion, there was a notable improvement in the patient's clinical condition
Dagtekin et al. [36]	Venlafaxine, Lamotrigine, Diazepam	Rigidity, hyperreflexia, and reflex myoclonia	2.5 mL/kg (150 mL) IV bolus of 20% lipid emulsion	8 h after admission in ICU	Symptoms improved after infusion started
Hillyard et al. [37]	Venlafaxine, Zopiclone	A decline in GCS to 3 points	1.5 mL/kg (100 mL) 20% lipid emulsion IV bolus dose followed by a 400 mL infusion over the next 40 min		30 min after infusion started, his GCS improved to 11 points and was 14 after 3 h
Blixt et al. [38]	Venlafaxine	Refractory cardiovascular collapse and PEA cardiac arrest	1.5 mL/kg 20% lipid emulsion IV bolus in 60 s followed by an infusion at a rate of 0.25 mL/kg/min over 60 min		No further PEA or cardiac arrest episodes occurred

There are a few studies that describe the effect of lower doses of ILE therapy, particularly in children. One case report described the successful treatment of quetiapine and citalopram overdose with the recommended bolus dosing, followed by a lower infusion dose of 0.025 mL/kg/min over 1 h [11]. Another case report illustrated the successful treatment of an overdose of quetiapine and fluvoxamine with a 1 mL/kg lipid emulsion bolus followed by a 0.05 mL/kg/min infusion for two hours [39].

The dosing regimen employed in our case was comparable to that utilized by other researchers. This approach resulted in a notable enhancement in clinical outcomes, prompting the decision to prolong the treatment duration for an additional two hours and to repeat the bolus dose when signs of cardiotoxicity reappeared. The administered medication did not exhibit any detrimental consequences, such as allergic responses, fat overload syndrome accompanied by hepatosplenomegaly, jaundice, acute pancreatitis, seizures, fat embolism, coagulopathies, or any alterations in laboratory test results.

After the acute problem is resolved, the patient may require psychological evaluation and treatment to address the root causes of the overdose and prevent future suicidal actions. Medication adjustments and/or hospitalization may be required for further evaluation and care of their mental health condition.

It is crucial to remember that the therapy for venlafaxine and quetiapine overdose can be complicated and may vary based on the patient's individual previous health status. As a result, it is critical to seek immediate medical assistance and consult with a skilled medical practitioner for advice on the best treatment approach.

4. Conclusions

This case report emphasizes the effective use of ILE therapy for severe cardiotoxicity induced by SSRI and antipsychotic overdose. We sustain that the potential utilization of lipid rescue therapy could go beyond its current role and function as a treatment for toxicity induced by local anesthetics.

In summary, despite possible adverse effects, lipid emulsion appears to have an evolving role in the management of a patient with a severe, life-threatening overdose of lipid-soluble compounds. It has been successfully used in the treatment of induced cardiotoxicity by severe overdoses with lipophilic drugs, such as quetiapine and venlafaxine. Overall, the use of intravenous lipid emulsion infusion for venlafaxine and quetiapine overdose needs further investigation. It may be considered as part of a comprehensive treatment plan, especially in those patients with severe cardiotoxicity refractory to maximum conventional therapy.

It should be noted, however, that the use of ILE infusion in drug overdose is still a relatively new and experimental therapy. Its safety and efficacy have not been thoroughly demonstrated. Therefore, it should only be used when the advantages outweigh the hazards and only under the supervision of a skilled medical expert.

Author Contributions: Conceptualization, C.C. and R.Ț.; methodology, L.M.; investigation, A.-M.C.; resources, R.U.; data curation, S.I.; writing—original draft preparation, C.-A.A.; writing—review and editing, C.C.; visualization, O.A.; supervision, I.M.G.; project administration, R.Ț.; funding acquisition, L.M. All authors have read and agreed to the published version of the manuscript.

Funding: This research received no external funding.

Institutional Review Board Statement: The study was conducted in accordance with the Declaration of Helsinki and approved by the Ethics Committee of the Clinical Emergency Hospital of Bucharest (protocol code 41144 and 3 October 2023) for studies involving humans.

Informed Consent Statement: Written informed consent was obtained from the patient to publish this paper.

Data Availability Statement: Data are contained within the article.

Conflicts of Interest: The authors declare no conflict of interest.

References

1. Schotte, A.; Janssen, P.F.M.; Gommeren, W.; Luyten, W.H.M.L.; Van Gompel, P.; Lesage, A.S.; De Loore, K.; Leysen, J.E. Risperidone compared with new and reference antipsychotic drugs: In vitro and in vivo receptor binding. *Psychopharmacology* **1996**, *124*, 57–73. [CrossRef]
2. Ngo, A.; Ciranni, M.; Olson, K.R. Acute Quetiapine Overdose in Adults: A 5-Year Retrospective Case Series. *Ann. Emerg. Med.* **2008**, *52*, 541–547. [CrossRef]
3. Holliday, S.M.; Benfield, P. Venlafaxine: A Review of its Pharmacology and Therapeutic Potential in Depression. *Drugs* **1995**, *49*, 280–294. [CrossRef]
4. Hawton, K.; Bergen, H.; Simkin, S.; Cooper, J.; Waters, K.; Gunnell, D.; Kapur, N. Toxicity of antidepressants: Rates of suicide relative to prescribing and non-fatal overdose. *Br. J. Psychiatry* **2010**, *196*, 354–358. [CrossRef] [PubMed]
5. Höjer, J.; Hulting, J.; Salmonson, H. Fatal cardiotoxicity induced by venlafaxine overdosage. *Clin. Toxicol.* **2008**, *46*, 336–337. [CrossRef]
6. Bosse, G.M.; Spiller, H.A.; Collins, A.M. A fatal case of venlafaxine overdose. *J. Med. Toxicol.* **2008**, *4*, 18–20. [CrossRef]
7. Howell, C.; Wilson, A.D.; Waring, W.S. Cardiovascular toxicity due to venlafaxine poisoning in adults: A review of 235 consecutive cases. *Br. J. Clin. Pharmacol.* **2007**, *64*, 192–197. [CrossRef] [PubMed]
8. Weinberg, G.L.; VadeBoncouer, T.; Ramaraju, G.A.; Garcia-Amaro, M.F.; Cwik, M.J. Pretreatment or Resuscitation with a Lipid Infusion Shifts the Dose-Response to Bupivacaine-induced Asystole in Rats. *Anesthesiology* **1998**, *88*, 1071–1075. [CrossRef]
9. Eren Cevik, S.; Tasyurek, T.; Guneysel, O. Intralipid emulsion treatment as an antidote in lipophilic drug intoxications. *Am. J. Emerg. Med.* **2014**, *32*, 1103–1108. [CrossRef]
10. Elgazzar, F.M.; Elgohary, M.S.; Basiouny, S.M.; Lashin, H.I. Intravenous lipid emulsion as an adjuvant therapy of acute clozapine poisoning. *Hum. Exp. Toxicol.* **2021**, *40*, 1053–1063. [CrossRef]
11. Purg, D.; Markota, A.; Grenc, D.; Sinkovič, A. Low-dose intravenous lipid emulsion for the treatment of severe quetiapine and citalopram poisoning. *Arh. Hig. Rada Toksikol.* **2016**, *67*, 164–166. [CrossRef] [PubMed]
12. Karcioglu, O. Use of lipid emulsion therapy in local anesthetic overdose. *Saudi Med. J.* **2017**, *38*, 985–993. [CrossRef] [PubMed]
13. Baud, F.J.; Megarbane, B.; Deye, N.; Leprince, P. Clinical review: Aggressive management and extracorporeal support for drug-induced cardiotoxicity. *Crit. Care* **2007**, *11*, 207. [CrossRef] [PubMed]
14. Pacher, P.; Kecskemeti, V. Cardiovascular Side Effects of New Antidepressants and Antipsychotics: New Drugs, old Concerns? *Curr. Pharm. Des.* **2005**, *10*, 2463–2475. [CrossRef]

15. Stoner, S.C. Management of serious cardiac adverse effects of antipsychotic medications. *Ment. Health Clin.* **2017**, *7*, 246–254. [CrossRef]
16. Neal, J.M.; Barrington, M.J.; Fettiplace, M.R.; Gitman, M.; Memtsoudis, S.G.; Mörwald, E.E.; Rubin, D.S.; Weinberg, G. The Third American Society of Regional Anesthesia and Pain Medicine Practice Advisory on Local Anesthetic Systemic Toxicity. *Obstet. Anesth. Dig.* **2018**, *38*, 171. [CrossRef]
17. Lavonas, E.J.; Drennan, I.R.; Gabrielli, A.; Heffner, A.C.; Hoyte, C.O.; Orkin, A.M.; Sawyer, K.N.; Donnino, M.W. Part 10: Special circumstances of resuscitation: 2015 American Heart Association guidelines update for cardiopulmonary resuscitation and emergency cardiovascular care. *Circulation* **2015**, *132* (Suppl. S2), S501–S518. [CrossRef]
18. Rothschild, L.; Bern, S.; Oswald, S.; Weinberg, G. Intravenous lipid emulsion in clinical toxicology. *Scand. J. Trauma. Resusc. Emerg. Med.* **2010**, *18*, 51. [CrossRef]
19. Fettiplace, M.R.; Weinberg, G. The Mechanisms Underlying Lipid Resuscitation Therapy. *Reg. Anesth. Pain Med.* **2018**, *43*, 138–149. [CrossRef]
20. Sepulveda, E.A.; Pak, A. Lipid Emulsion Therapy. In *StatPearls*; StatPearls Publishing: St. Petersburg, FL, USA, 2023. Available online: https://www.ncbi.nlm.nih.gov/books/NBK549897 (accessed on 6 November 2023).
21. Kuo, I.; Akpa, B.S. Validity of the lipid sink as a mechanism for the reversal of local anesthetic systemic toxicity: A physiologically based pharmacokinetic model study. *Anesthesiology* **2013**, *118*, 1350–1361. [CrossRef]
22. Partownavid, P.; Umar, S.; Li, J.; Rahman, S.; Eghbali, M. Fatty-acid oxidation and calcium homeostasis are involved in the rescue of bupivacaine-induced cardiotoxicity by lipid emulsion in rats. *Crit. Care Med.* **2012**, *40*, 2431–2437. [CrossRef] [PubMed]
23. Stehr, S.N.; Ziegeler, J.C.; Pexa, A.; Oertel, R.; Deussen, A.; Koch, T.; Hübler, M. The effects of lipid infusion on myocardial function and bioenergetics in L-bupivacaine toxicity in the isolated rat heart. *Anesth. Analg.* **2007**, *104*, 186–192. [CrossRef]
24. Gosselin, S.; Hoegberg, L.C.G.; Hoffman, R.S.; Graudins, A.; Stork, C.M.; Thomas, S.H.L.; Stellpflug, S.J.; Hayes, B.D.; Levine, M.; Morris, M.; et al. Evidence-based recommendations on the use of intravenous lipid emulsion therapy in poisoning. *Clin. Toxicol.* **2016**, *54*, 899–923. [CrossRef] [PubMed]
25. Jaffal, K.; Chevillard, L.; Mégarbane, B. Lipid Emulsion to Treat Acute Poisonings: Mechanisms of Action, Indications, and Controversies. *Pharmaceutics* **2023**, *15*, 1396. [CrossRef] [PubMed]
26. Cave, G.; Harvey, M.G. Should we consider the infusion of lipid emulsion in the resuscitation of poisoned patients? *Crit. Care* **2014**, *18*, 457. [CrossRef] [PubMed]
27. Nedialkov, A.M.; Umadhay, T.; Valdes, J.A.; Campbell, Y. Intravenous Fat Emulsion for Treatment of Local Anesthetic Systemic Toxicity: Best Practice and Review of the Literature. *AANA J.* **2018**, *86*, 290–297. [PubMed]
28. Sirianni, A.J.; Osterhoudt, K.C.; Calello, D.P.; Muller, A.A.; Waterhouse, M.R.; Goodkin, M.B.; Weinberg, G.L.; Henretig, F.M. Use of Lipid Emulsion in the Resuscitation of a Patient With Prolonged Cardiovascular Collapse After Overdose of Bupropion and Lamotrigine. *Ann. Emerg. Med.* **2008**, *51*, 412–415. [CrossRef]
29. Oti, C.; Uncles, D.; Sable, N.; Willers, J. The use of Intralipid for unconsciousness after a mixed overdose. *Anaesthesia* **2009**, *65*, 110–111. [CrossRef]
30. Finn, S.D.H.; Uncles, D.R.; Willers, J.; Sable, N. Early treatment of a quetiapine and sertraline overdose with Intralipid®. *Anaesthesia* **2009**, *64*, 191–194. [CrossRef]
31. Bartos, M.; Knudsen, K. Use of intravenous lipid emulsion in the resuscitation of a patient with cardiovascular collapse after a severe overdose of quetiapine. *Clin. Toxicol.* **2013**, *51*, 501–504. [CrossRef] [PubMed]
32. Arslan, E.D.; Demir, A.; Yilmaz, F.; Kavalci, C.; Karakilic, E.; Çelikel, E. Treatment of quetiapine overdose with intravenous lipid emulsion. *Keio J. Med.* **2013**, *62*, 53–57. [CrossRef] [PubMed]
33. Hieger, M.A.; Peters, N.E. Lipid Emulsion Therapy for Quetiapine Overdose. *Am. J. Ther.* **2020**, *27*, E518–E519. [CrossRef]
34. Harvey, M.; Cave, G. Case report: Successful lipid resuscitation in multidrug overdose with predominant tricyclic antidepressant toxidrome. *Int. J. Emerg. Med.* **2012**, *5*, 8. [CrossRef] [PubMed]
35. de Wit, D.; Franssen, E.J.F.; Verstoep, N. Intralipid administration in case of a severe venlafaxine overdose in a patient with previous gastric bypass surgery. *Toxicol. Rep.* **2022**, *9*, 1139–1141. [CrossRef] [PubMed]
36. Dagtekin, O.; Marcus, H.; Müller, C.; Böttiger, B.W.; Spöhr, F. Lipid therapy for serotonin syndrome after intoxication with venlafaxine, lamotrigine and diazepam. *Minerva Anestesiol.* **2011**, *77*, 93–95.
37. Hillyard, S.G.; Barrera-Groba, C.; Tighe, R. Intralipid reverses coma associated with zopiclone and venlafaxine overdose. *Eur. J. Anaesthesiol.* **2010**, *27*, 582–583. [CrossRef] [PubMed]
38. John, B.; Shazia, R.; Stephen, B. Severe Venlafaxine Intoxication with Refractory Pulseless Electrical Activity Cardiac Arrest Successfully Treated with Intravenous Lipid Emulsion. *Int. J. Crit. Care Emerg. Med.* **2018**, *4*, 44. [CrossRef]
39. Hubbard, A.M.; House, L.M.; Lee, J.M. Low-dose lipid emulsion for pediatric vasoplegic shock due to quetiapine and fluvoxamine overdose: A case report. *J. Emerg. Crit. Care Med.* **2022**, *6*, 28. [CrossRef]

Disclaimer/Publisher's Note: The statements, opinions and data contained in all publications are solely those of the individual author(s) and contributor(s) and not of MDPI and/or the editor(s). MDPI and/or the editor(s) disclaim responsibility for any injury to people or property resulting from any ideas, methods, instructions or products referred to in the content.

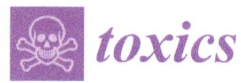

Review

Quetiapine-Related Deaths: In Search of a Surrogate Endpoint

Ivan Šoša

Department of Anatomy, Faculty of Medicine, University of Rijeka, 51000 Rijeka, Croatia; ivan.sosa@uniri.hr

Abstract: Quetiapine is a second-generation antipsychotic drug available for two and half decades. Due to increased misuse, prescription outside the approved indications, and availability on the black market, it is being encountered in medicolegal autopsies more frequently. For instance, it has been linked to increased mortality rates, most likely due to its adverse effects on the cardiovascular system. Its pharmacokinetic features and significant postmortem redistribution challenge traditional sampling in forensic toxicology. Therefore, a systematic literature review was performed, inclusive of PubMed, the Web of Science—core collection, and the Scopus databases; articles were screened for the terms "quetiapine", "death", and "autopsy" to reevaluate each matrix used as a surrogate endpoint in the forensic toxicology of quetiapine-related deaths. Ultimately, this review considers the results of five studies that were well presented (more than two matrices, data available for all analyses, for instance). The highest quetiapine concentrations were usually measured in the liver tissue. As interpreted by their authors, the results of the considered studies showed a strong correlation between some matrices, but, unfortunately, the studies presented models with poor goodness of fit. The distribution of quetiapine in distinct body compartments/tissues showed no statistically significant relationship with the length of the postmortem interval. Furthermore, this study did not confirm the anecdotal correlation of peripheral blood concentrations with skeletal muscle concentrations. Otherwise, there was no consistency regarding selecting an endpoint for analysis.

Keywords: forensic toxicology; quetiapine; relevant matrix; tissue modeling

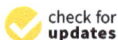

Citation: Šoša, I. Quetiapine-Related Deaths: In Search of a Surrogate Endpoint. *Toxics* **2024**, *12*, 37. https://doi.org/10.3390/toxics12010037

Academic Editor: Hartmut W. Jaeschke

Received: 20 November 2023
Revised: 30 December 2023
Accepted: 1 January 2024
Published: 3 January 2024

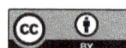

Copyright: © 2024 by the author. Licensee MDPI, Basel, Switzerland. This article is an open access article distributed under the terms and conditions of the Creative Commons Attribution (CC BY) license (https://creativecommons.org/licenses/by/4.0/).

1. Introduction

Quetiapine is an atypical antipsychotic drug (a second-generation antipsychotic drug) used to treat schizophrenia, bipolar, borderline personality, and major depressive disorders; broadly speaking, this treatment has numerous neurocognitive, neuroprotective, and potential off-label indications [1,2]. Developed in 1985, the US approved quetiapine for medical use in 1997; now, it is on the World Health Organization's List of Essential Medicines [3,4]. Regarding the non-approved uses of approved drugs, the most frequent such use for quetiapine is its wide use as a sleep aid due to its sedating effects [5,6]. The benefits of off-label use do not appear to outweigh the side effects. Nevertheless, it is reported to treat conditions such as Tourette's syndrome, musical hallucinations, etc. [7–9]. Unlike most other antipsychotics, its hypnotic and sedative effects offset any problems with patient compliance.

Quetiapine' appears to have low dopamine receptor affinity and intense antihistamine activity, which renders it similar to sedating antihistamines [10]. Approximately 90% of serotonin in the human body is stored in the gastrointestinal tract, and quetiapine has a moderate affinity for its receptors [11]. Notwithstanding, quetiapine shows an affinity for various neurotransmitter receptors [12]. Not only does it enhance the serotoninergic transmission, but serotonin, a key neurotransmitter of the brain–gut axis, also plays a vital role in the pathogenesis of emotional distress and gastrointestinal diseases [13]. Specifically, it binds serotonin (5-hydroxytryptamine; 5HT) 5HT2A, adrenergic (α1), muscarinic, and histaminergic receptors, and it has a relatively weak affinity for dopamine D2 receptors [14,15], with an occupancy half-life about twice as long as that for plasma. All of these are cell-surface receptors that intervene in cellular communication.

For quetiapine toxicity to be fatal, it is necessary to combine it with other drugs [16]. Acute overdose typically results in sedation or hypotension and tachycardia, but cardiac arrhythmias, coma, and death have also been reported [17]. For some of them, severe overdosage may result in seizures requiring intubation/mechanical ventilation.

Some cases are hallmarked by cardiac and sinus tachycardia [18–20]. Generally, 10–25 mg/L levels are observed in the blood samples obtained from fatal cases during postmortem examinations. Non-toxic levels in postmortem blood extend to around 0.8 mg/kg, but, at the same time, toxic levels in postmortem blood can begin at 0.35 mg/kg. The serum or plasma of quetiapine overdose survivors had concentrations ranging from 1 to 10 mg/L [21–23].

Even though the blockage of histamine-1 receptors produces the soothing effect of quetiapine, arrhythmogenic effects result from the channel inhibition of the ether-a-go-go-related gene (hERG). This may influence the QT interval [24]. The presence of some cardiovascular pathologies, for example, coronary disease, could be the lethal trigger if quetiapine is used, as seen in polydrug intoxications [25,26]. Quetiapine's deadly effect is governed by whether some medication potentiates this inhibition effect and, if so, to what extent [27,28]. As for respiratory depression, Culebras et al. reported its incidence in three patients on combined antipsychotic–opioid therapy [29]. In randomized clinical trials (RCTs) involving humans, considering the interactions of first-generation antipsychotics and morphine, sedation was scored on a sedation score tool. In eight of the fourteen RCTs, increased sedation scores were reported when morphine and droperidol were combined [19,27]. After the drug's ingestion and its rapid absorption, it reaches the maximum plasma concentration after 1.5 h, where it binds mostly (83%) to non-specific plasma proteins (human albumin) [13,15,30]. Quetiapine's bioavailability depends mainly on its first-pass metabolism, which is as poor as 9% [31,32]. Notably, the liver metabolizes many drugs, resulting in the production of water-soluble compounds that can be excreted via the bile [33]. In one stage, this process relies upon the "phase 1 reactions" mediated by cytochrome p450 (CYP). Oxidation, reduction, and hydrolysis reactions are mainly directed by the CYP isozyme CYP3A4. This explains why any drug interaction that modifies quetiapine's metabolism and pharmacokinetics is more likely to occur with drugs that are inhibitors or inducers of CYP3A4, rather than inhibitors of CYP2D6.

Bearing all of this in mind, this systematic review of the literature aims to identify studies with sufficient laboratory data to identify an alternative matrix to be used in the forensic investigation of quetiapine-related deaths.

2. Use and Misuse

In a formal sense, issues related to the misuse and abuse potential of quetiapine have not been regarded as a danger. However, those who administer quetiapine should be cautious when prescribing it to individuals with a history of substance abuse (particularly with opioids or anxiolytics). These individuals are "loose cannons" and are at increased risk.

Typically, people whose deaths are related to quetiapine are men in their mid-forties. Their leading causes of death at this age are drug toxicity and natural diseases. Less frequently, however, these deaths are linked to physical assaults [17].

Occasionally, quetiapine is associated with drug misuse, but it has limited potential for misuse [34]. Misuse is most often seen in patients with a history of polysubstance abuse and/or mental illness (especially those who are detained in prisons or secure psychiatric institutions) because the limited access to alternative intoxicants brings quetiapine to the fore.

However, quetiapine has been found to be associated with drug-seeking behavior more than any other atypical antipsychotic. It has standardized street prices and slang terms, such as "Q-ball" (referring to the intravenous injection of quetiapine mixed with cocaine), either alone or in combination with other drugs [16,19].

Quetiapine-Related Fatalities and Fatal Toxicity

Due to increased misuse and availability on the black market, quetiapine-associated deaths are frequently seen in medicolegal practice. Unintentional self-poisoning fatalities are classically related to substance abuse, mental health issues, and physical health problems; quetiapine is no exception. Fatalities—complex suicides and suicide attempts involving antipsychotic or sedative–hypnotic medications are frequently seen [35–37]. Poisoning homicides are rare, though they have been described, and quetiapine is used only to incapacitate the victim (as in pediatric homicides) [16,38,39].

Some reports on quetiapine-related deaths and series lack clinical details or provide only single quetiapine serum concentrations rather than a kinetic course. However, increasing numbers of studies provide more detailed clinical and analytical data on severe overdose cases. Available data from 1998 to 2021 in England and Wales could be a helpful introduction to the field. In Figure 1, six hundred ninety-six deaths involving quetiapine were presented [40]. A similar, increasing trend of misuse, non-fatal, and fatal overdoses was registered in Victoria (Australia) in the study (2006–2016) conducted by Lee et al. [41]. Mortality data from the European Union are not available

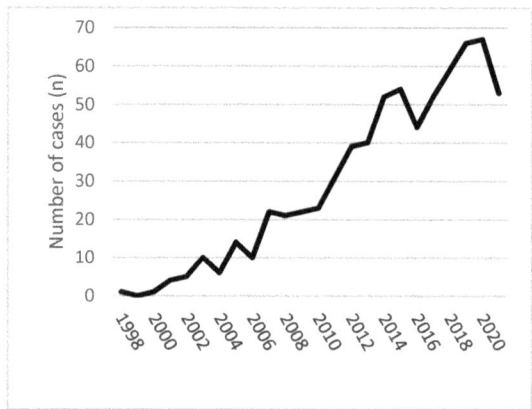

Figure 1. Quetiapine-related mortality in England and Wales 1998–2021 [40].

Kales et al. provided estimates of the direct mortality risk over 180 days, comparing individual antipsychotic agents and valproic acid. The mortality risk was found to vary, ranging from quetiapine (lowest) to haloperidol (highest). In fact, quetiapine use had the lowest effect on mortality, with a 3.2% (95% CI = 1.6–4.9%; $p < 0.01$) higher mortality risk than antidepressants (31; 95% CI = 21–62) [42,43].

As reported by Breivik et al., a Norwegian cohort showed no clear relationship for the length of the postmortem interval [44]. Their study showed that the postmortem interval was weakly correlated (positive correlation) with the quetiapine concentration in peripheral blood (mg/L). Moreover, the regression model was invalid ($p = 0.27$) with poor goodness of fit ($R2 = 0.16$). The same was found for central blood, brain, muscle, and liver tissue. This result agreed with the study of Vignali et al., where a weak positive correlation of postmortem interval was noted only for liver tissue [45]. When the post-mortem interval has been so long that extensively putrefied bodies are assessed, the analysis of entomological samples may support and complement the toxicological results [46]. Even in the case of dried blood spots, the quantification of quetiapine is possible with good recovery rates, within the concentration range of 0.05–1.0 µg/mL [47].

3. A Systematic Review Strategy and a Meta-Analysis

This study used a systematic literature review based on PRISMA guidelines to assess the postmortem management of quetiapine-related deaths (Figure 2) [48,49]. The term "quetiapine-related death" refers to deaths where quetiapine was linked to the cause of death anywhere in the causal chain. The literature is abundant in such cases; they are either complex suicides or homicides (where quetiapine was the reason for sedation/incapacitation), accidental intoxications, or polydrug overdoses.

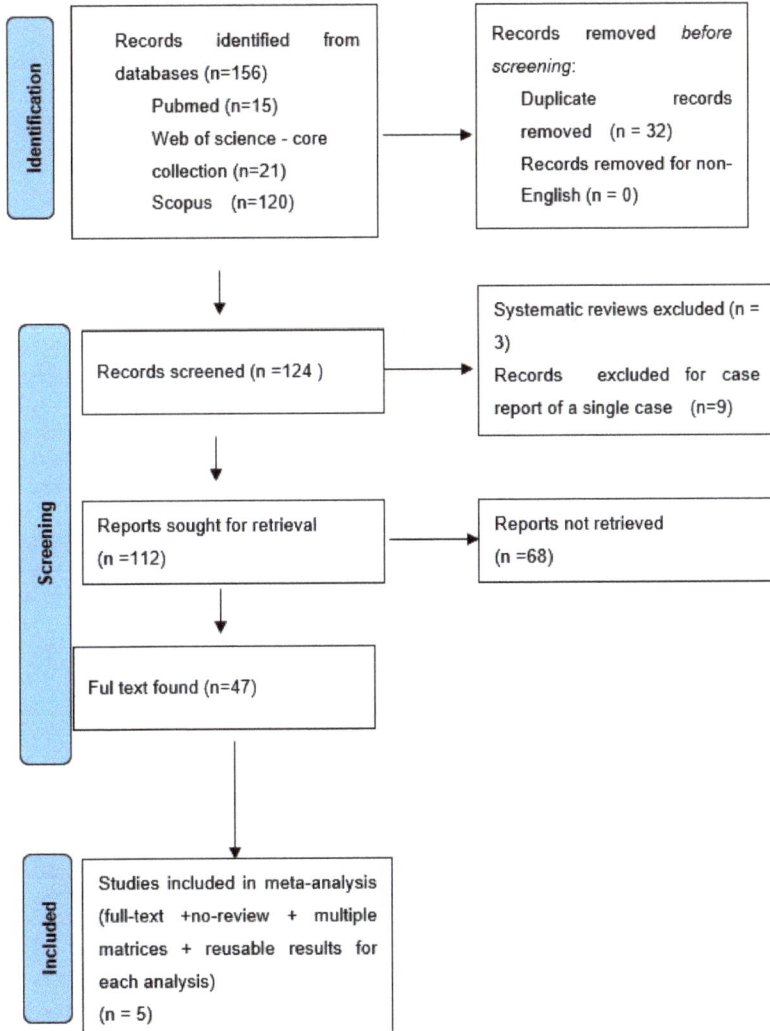

Figure 2. Methodology of literature search—systematic review according to the PRISMA guidelines [49].

Starting from their inception, PubMed, Web of Science—core collection, and the Scopus databases were screened for "quetiapine" AND "death" AND "autopsy." After finding 156 records, 32 duplicates were eliminated after being found using the automated bibliography tool. Finally, three systematic reviews, and nine case reports of a single case, were eliminated. Such an approach resulted in 112 entries (English language, "no-single case "case report, original papers, literature reviews, and meta-analyses), of which 47 full texts were available. Five researchers listed in Table 1. involving post-analytical results obtained from multiple matrices were included in the meta-analysis and discussed in this paper (therefore, were inclusion/exclusion criteria).

Table 1. Characteristics of the included studies.

Study	Year	Participants	Method	Interventions	Correction of the Measurement Units
Anderson and Fritz [50]	2000	7	Experimental case series	Postmortem toxicology	no
Hopenwasser et al. [51]	2004	8	Experimental case series	Postmortem toxicology	no
Parker and McIntyre [18]	2005	21	Experimental case series	Postmortem toxicology	no
Vignali et al. [45]	2020	13	Experimental case series	Postmortem toxicology	yes
Breivik et al. [44]	2020	14	Experimental case series	Postmortem toxicology	no

The meta-analysis correlation of blood quetiapine with other matrices lacks a marked significance level (p-value). In cases where this was missing, the correlation could not be proved, so this was considered to be incomplete outcome data (attrition bias, Figure 3). The same was the case in the absence of a marked control cohort. Studies by Anderson and Fritz [50] and Vignali et al. [45] have the form of case reports, even though they do present several cases (Table 1), so this is considered a risk of selection bias (random sequence generation issue). The reason for this problem lies in the practice of forensic pathologists (and all forensic toxicologists are either pathologists or are related closely to forensic pathologists) to rely on experience and individual customary practice in formulating their opinions is a potential source of low goodness of fit or statistically insignificant results in some cases. Conversely, case reports play a critical role in defining new entities, applying toxicological expertise, and obtaining data that other researchers could not accept due to regulations Not considering "post-mortem factors" was considered an "other bias" issue.

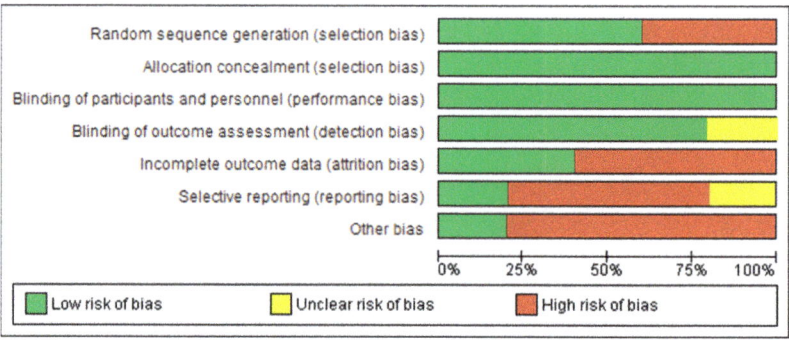

Figure 3. Risk of bias graph for studies included in meta-analysis: review authors' judgments about each risk of bias item presented as percentages across all included studies.

4. Relevant Matrices

Out of five studies included in this meta-analysis, 238 toxicological analyses involving 63 postmortems were performed. Although analyses were performed on a series of different matrices, those that were most frequently used (and are more traditional) are given in Figure 4.

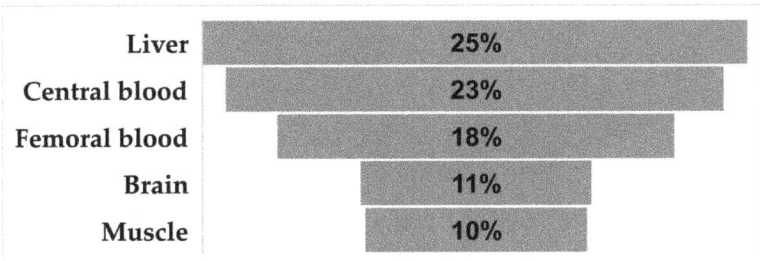

Figure 4. Matrices used in >10% of cases.

4.1. The Liver and Its Lobar Structure

The liver is a highly vascularized, large (typically weighing around 1.5 kg), and encapsulated organ situated to a large extent in the upper right front portion of the abdomen. It is divided into two major lobes; the smaller left lobe partially overlays the ventricle [52,53].

The left lobe is smaller and more flattened than the right. Its undersurface presents a gastric impression and omental tuberosity. Brevik et al. prepared a report of seven participants (7/14, 50%) from whom paired samples of liver tissue were obtained (both lobes). A paired t-test of two samples for means established no significant difference regarding quetiapine accumulation in either lobe. The left liver lobe is most likely more susceptible than the right lobe to the postmortem redistribution of zopiclone, and some of its constituents are thinner due to its anatomical proximity to the stomach (see Table 2) [54,55]. The documented postmortem redistribution of the drug from the biliary system can also contribute to its apparent accumulation in hepatic tissue [44,56,57]. Classic biliary anatomy includes the left hepatic duct, which emerges from the umbilical fissure along the inferior border of the left lobe. The right hepatic duct drains the right liver lobe and comprises two major branches, the right posterior duct and the right anterior duct [58].

Table 2. Table of correlations and a goodness of fit for quetiapine concentrations in liver tissue vs. bile or stomach content.

Study	Year	Pearson Correlation Coefficient (r)	R2 (Goodness of Fit)	p-Value	Matrix
Anderson and Fritz [50]	2000	0.21	0.04	0.22	Bile
Anderson and Fritz [50]	2000	0.51	0.26	0.02	Gastric content
Hopenwasser et al. [51]	2004	0.99	0.97	0.19	Bile
Hopenwasser et al. [51]	2004	−0.33	0.11	0.23	Gastric content
Parker and McIntyre [18]	2005	−0.15	0.02	0.04	Gastric content
Vignali et al. [45]	2020	0.52	0.28	0.0005	Bile

4.2. First-Pass Effect and the Liver

The liver is the body's primary site for drug metabolism and contains the largest quantity of the critical cytochrome enzyme system, liver alcohol dehydrogenase, and many other enzymes. Like most xenobiotics, including drugs, quetiapine's pharmacology and toxicology are largely inextricably linked to its metabolism. Due to its significant metabolic potential, central anatomical position, and ability to take away chemicals from the blood, the liver constitutes an organ with a high susceptibility to the effects of xenobiotics. The liver's involvement is the most obvious in transaminase elevations. These typically occur by the third week of treatment, and levels return to baseline with continued quetiapine administration [56].

The drug's volume of distribution while it spreads throughout the body is 10 ± 4 Ukg [15,50]. Quetiapine is orally administered as a fumarate salt in the form of tablets. Daily doses in adults range from 150 to 750 mg, and steady-state concentrations are achieved within two days of dosing [59]. No specific plasma proteins that carry quetiapine were identified; however, it is converted into the active proteins and metabolites norquetiapine and 7-hydroxy quetiapine [60,61]. Both were assessed in patients autopsied in the study of Vignali et al. The authors found (peripheral) blood levels of norquetiapine to be 258.93 (95% CI = −22.63–540.48). Blood levels of 7-hydroxy quetiapine were 45.88 (95% CI = −8.24–83.52) [22,45].

The cytochrome P450 (CYP) system has been observed to extensively metabolize quetiapine in the liver, with less than 5% of the original drug appearing in urine (and minimally in other excretions). Around 73% of 150mg of quetiapine radiolabeled with 100 mCi ^{14}C was recovered in the urine and 21% in the feces within 168 h of administration. The mean terminal half-life of quetiapine is about six hours; in its unchanged form, it accounted for less than 1% of the excreted substance [15,62].

Though quetiapine is excreted with urine, it has a low renal elimination rate (less than 5%) and a relatively large volume of distribution (Vd = 10 l/kg), so forced diuresis is no longer recommended [63,64]. The elimination half-life can be easily calculated as follows:

As assessed in several case series, the concentration level of quetiapine was noticeably higher in the liver tissue than in any other postmortem sample [18,44,50]. This paradigm was most evident in the study of Parker and McIntyre (16.09 (CI 95% = 4.96–27.22) mg/kg). However, the linear regression model showed no statistical significance (the p-value was 0.09). Anderson and Fritz showed a more distinct and statistically significant positive correlation of quetiapine concentrations between the peripheral blood and liver tissue (R^2 = 0.99; p = 0.01), although their study consisted of only five participants who were eligible for the linear regression model (27.86 (CI 95% = −31.05 to 86.77 mg/kg)). Another study that assessed quetiapine concentrations in eight liver samples reported 5.11 (CI 95% = 1.11–9.11 mg/kg) [51]. In this regard, the study that included the most sizable cohort was that of Vignali et al. from 2020. It comprised 12 liver samples with mean quetiapine concentrations of 1002.9811 (CI 95% = 57.64–1948.32 mg/kg) [45].

4.3. Liver Tissue from Fresh Cadavers

Resected liver biopsies can be sliced with retained original cellular diversity and in vivo cellular architecture. They can be cultured ex vivo for two weeks [65,66]. Routine toxicology is performed on these tissues using mass spectrometry (GC-MS) or specific high-pressure liquid chromatography (HPLC) [30,67]. Both methods are relatively sensitive, with a limit of quantification for HPLC of µg/L, and the GC-MS method is accurate to 2 µg/L [15] (see Table 3).

Table 3. Correlation and goodness of fit for peripheral blood and liver tissue.

Study	Year	Pearson Correlation Coefficient (r)	R^2 (Goodness of Fit)	p-Value
Anderson and Fritz [50]	2000	0.82	0.68	0.23
Hopenwasser et al. [51]	2004	−0.28	0.08	0.94
Parker and McIntyre [18]	2005	0.37	0.14	0.04
Breivik et al. [44]	2020	0.82	0.66	0.27
Vignali et al. [45]	2020	−0.26	0.07	0.25

4.4. Liver Tissue Modeling

Normal hepatocytes, constituting nearly 60% of the total cell population within the liver, along with the HepaRG cell line, are capable of performing the majority of liver functions, including many drug-processing activities at various levels [68]. Transcribing liver-specific genes at high levels without fresh human tissue is challenging, but it can even provide differentiated hepatocyte-like HepaRG cells. In fact, it is more successful than any other liver cell line. As HepaRG cells express most of the drug-processing genes, including major CYPs and UGTs, it should not be surprising that these cell lines have been used as pharmacological and toxicological models [68–70]. According to Le Daré et al., a higher quetiapine metabolism was observed in differentiated HepaRG cells (50% of quetiapine metabolized) compared to pHH (25% of quetiapine metabolized) [71–73]. This helps meet the desired feature of human cell models, stably expressing the functional properties of the in vivo cells they are derived from in order to predict the toxicity of chemicals [74]. Indeed, in vitro models of human liver preparations seem to be the most lucrative models with maximum feasibility. Cellular and subcellular systems are included in these models, and they can equally contain HepG2 and HuH7 hepatic cell lines (developed from liver tumors and preserved hepatocytes) [74–76]. The primary functional cells of the liver, the hepatocytes, have historically been challenging to culture ex vivo. Various complementary in vitro liver models have been introduced to overcome this difficulty. These models are classically categorized into 2D and 3D models. At the same time, none are simple and effective for predicting all hepatic functions (specifically, the clearance of chemicals).

Even though 2D models are flexible, affordable, and valuable for studies that require large numbers of cells, most cell lines do not have normal liver-specific functions, including those relevant to toxicology. They are genetically abnormal and do not adequately reproduce hepatocyte biology. Meanwhile, 3D cultures offer cell–cell and cell–extracellular matrix interactions, though these methods are often more challenging to translate into high-throughput tactics. Primary hepatocytes in 3D modeling can form spheroids, prolonging the maintenance of hepatic phenotype and function. The ability to transiently proliferate and self-organize is a well-known ability of hepatic cells, and it has also been taken advantage of in forming liver organoids. Organoid models have been developed from various hepatic cell types, and all exhibit various degrees of similarity to human hepatocytes [66,77,78]. Hepatocytes with or without non-parenchymal cells can be spatially patterned in 3D, using, for instance, soft lithography. Combining 3D printing technologies with cytocompatible biological "inks" enables engineers to bioprint tissue models, incorporating parenchymal and stromal cells in spatially patterned arrangements. Unfortunately, such "futuristic" models are challenging to make and maintain.

Since in vivo quetiapine metabolism pathways generate well-defined metabolite derivatives, this drug was used to explore the consistency of the in vitro metabolic model. Out of many emerging preclinical human-relevant in vitro models used to evaluate toxic injury to the liver, in silico modeling has shown good potential in terms of its affordability and easy maintenance [68]. Mathematical modeling, referred to as physiologically based pharmacokinetic (PBPK) modeling, is basically an in silico technique where mathematical modeling is used to inform and optimize the design in, for instance, forensic toxicology [79]. In the same context, forensic toxicologists should benefit from the estimated time course concentrations [80]. Reported human blood concentrations of quetiapine were considered in the context of the environment that includes the receptor (gut), metabolizing agent (liver), and central compartments with blood-to-plasma concentration ratios (Rb) and liver-to-plasma concentration ratios (Kp,h) [81,82]. Alternatively, some other compounds may be estimated using in silico tools. All of these are important clinical parameters for calculating pharmacokinetic (PK) properties [83]. In recent years, there has been significant progress in developing liver-emulating technologies, including liver-on-a-chip. Biochemical and metabolic information is chip-generated [84]. However, this advanced and highly sensitive technology is still in its infancy, as methodologies, procedures, and standards render the obtained data difficult to handle in the grossing room or in medicolegal settings in general [85].

4.5. Blood

Since the drug's blood level is the one that affects the individual, blood is the most important tissue for toxicological analysis. This accounts for central (e.g., heart) and peripheral (e.g., femoral) blood. Although there are cases where peripheral vs. central blood concentrations differed significantly, none of the five included studies showed significant differences between the endpoints (*p*-values varied from 0.18 to 0.59; for overall effect see Figure 5). The results from previous studies indicate that drug concentrations in the central blood are generally higher than in the peripheral blood [86].

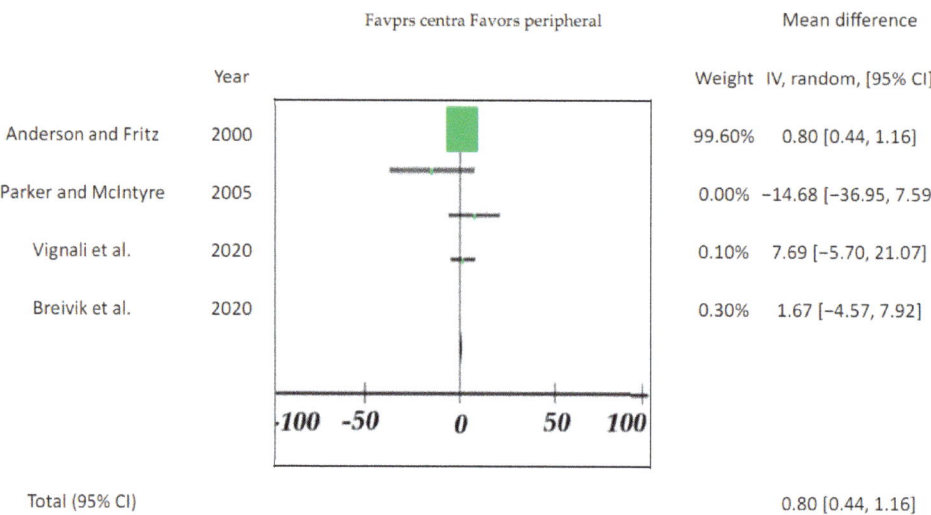

Figure 5. Forest plot of comparison of different blood matrices. For four studies that considered central and peripheral blood, pooled variance (Sp2) was calculated at 245.89 ng/mL with a pooled standard deviation of ±15.68 [18,44,45,50].

4.6. Brain Tissue

Several studies considered brain tissue's quetiapine, and in the study of Breivik et al. this concentration correlated moderately (positive correlation) with that in the peripheral blood ($r = 0.5$); unfortunately, the linear regression model was below the level of statistical significance [44]. Skov et al. even claim brain concentrations are about four times those in the blood [87] (see Table 4 containing data reviewed here).

Table 4. Table of correlations and goodness of fit for quetiapine concentrations in peripheral blood vs. brain tissue.

Study	Year	Pearson Correlation Coefficient (r)	R2 (Goodness of Fit)	*p*-Value
Hopenwasser et al. [51]	2004	Only two samples	0.19	
Breivik et al. [44]	2020	0.50	0.25	0.24
Vignali et al. [45]	2020	0.05	0.002	0.25

4.7. Skeletal Muscle

Breivik et al. even concluded that, in the absence of blood, skeletal muscle may be treated as a preferred matrix for quetiapine concentrations since its concentration in skeletal muscle correlated well with that in peripheral blood. Hopenwasser et al.'s related data indicate a strong positive correlation between blood and skeletal muscle quetiapine concentrations. Their study participants showed $r = 0.98$ in a linear model with $R^2 = 0.97$. Unfortunately, the *p*-value was, likewise, inappropriate at 0.07 [51]. A strong positive correlation (r = 0.92) was obtained in a linear model with a *p*-value of 0.98. The same was true in the cohort of Vignali et al. in which a strong correlation was obtained for a poor model (r = 0.80, R2 = 0.63, *p*-value = 0.51) [44,45]. Nevertheless, quetiapine's implication in the metabolism of lipids in the skeletal muscle is visible in lipidomics [88].

In conclusion, Burghardt et al.'s findings suggest that atypical antipsychotics change the lipid profiles of human skeletal muscle, so the role of that tissue in quetiapine metabolism should be assessed in the future [62,88]. Precisely because of this, it should be no surprise that Breivik et al. (b) validated the method for determining quetiapine in postmortem skeletal tissue [89].

5. Other Matrices

The blood, the brain, the liver, and the muscle tissue were all used as preferred matrices in those five studies of interest to this review. Of 238 samples assessed, 59 (24.79%) were liver tissue. Blood, as a primary tissue of toxicological interest, whether central or peripheral, was considered in 54/238 (22.59%) and 43/238 (18.07%) cases, respectively. Brain and skeletal muscle were both bordering on 10% of cases. The brain was assessed in 25/238 (10.5%), and the skeletal muscle in 247/38 (10.1%).

Other less frequently used matrices are given in Figure 6.

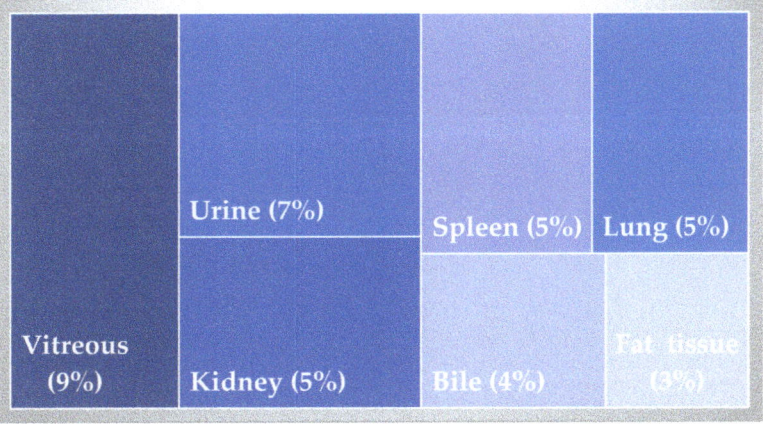

Figure 6. Less frequently used matrices.

Pathologists' choices seem unfortunate since bile and vitreous are traditionally preferred matrices in forensic toxicology [90]. More so considering moderate positive correlations of femoral blood's quetiapine and the concentrations of quetiapine in vitreous or bile. However, peripheral blood's quetiapine and its concentrations in vitreous correlated (though weakly) in the study of (r = 0.32, R^2 = 0.11, *p*-value = 0.04) [18]. Vignali et al. correlated bile with peripheral blood more straightforwardly (r = 0.52, R^2 = 0.28, *p*-value = 0.01) [45].

Lastly, quetiapine concentrations in hair segments have been assessed. Such an assessment is a step forward in therapeutic drug monitoring. Not counting the practical significance of this endpoint in forensic toxicology. Unfortunately, none of the five studies considered included hair concentrations of quetiapine, so more detailed calculations are unavailable. For the completeness of this review, note that several studies have been published over the years on antipsychotics in hair, and quetiapine is not an exception. Studies also report quetiapine concentrations in nails [91–94]. Nevertheless, nails should be preferred as a relevant matrix since they retain certain substances more likely to have concentrations than hair [95,96].

6. Conclusions

When blood is not available, the analysis of other tissues can provide important information that helps diagnose potential intoxication with quetiapine. The search for an adequate alternative endpoint seems rational, considering the increasing trend of quetiapine misuse and overdoses.

The relatively high concentrations of quetiapine in the liver tissue, and the modest (if any) statistical significance when correlating other endpoints with blood, cast a suspicion on any straightforward recommendation for selecting a relevant matrix. Further investigations and the integration of results obtained in silico and in vitro are needed to improve routine forensic toxicology. Recent endeavors where hair or nails were used as surrogate endpoints point out the advantages of keratin matrices that are much more resistant to post-mortem decomposition than other biological samples. Even though the evidence on the feasibility of keratinized matrices in this regard is missing, these reports could answer this paper's query.

Funding: This research received no external funding.

Institutional Review Board Statement: Not applicable.

Informed Consent Statement: Not applicable.

Data Availability Statement: Available on request.

Acknowledgments: This author acknowledges the University of Rijeka, Faculty of Medicine, for its constant support. The author also acknowledges efforts of the Croatian Institute of Public Health.

Conflicts of Interest: The funders had no role in the design of the study; in the collection, analyses, or interpretation of data; in the writing of the manuscript; or in the decision to publish the results.

References

1. Soeiro, D.E.S.M.G.; Dias, V.V.; Missio, G.; Balanza-Martinez, V.; Valiengo, L.; Carvalho, A.F.; Moreno, R.A. Role of quetiapine beyond its clinical efficacy in bipolar disorder: From neuroprotection to the treatment of psychiatric disorders (Review). *Exp. Ther. Med.* **2015**, *9*, 643–652. [CrossRef]
2. Morrison, P.; Taylor, D.M.; McGuire, P. Schizophrenia and Related Psychoses. In *The Maudsley Prescribing Guidelines in Psychiatry*; John Wiley & Sons: Hoboken, NJ, USA, 2021; pp. 1–224.
3. World Health Organization (WHO). *WHO Model List of Essential Medicines-22nd List*; WHO: Geneva, Switzerland, 2021.
4. Curry, D.E.; Richards, B.L. A Brief Review of Quetiapine. *Am. J. Psychiatry Resid. J.* **2022**, *18*, 20–22. [CrossRef]
5. Lin, C.Y.; Chiang, C.H.; Tseng, M.M.; Tam, K.W.; Loh, E.W. Effects of quetiapine on sleep: A systematic review and meta-analysis of clinical trials. *Eur. Neuropsychopharmacol.* **2023**, *67*, 22–36. [CrossRef]
6. Anderson, S.L.; Vande Griend, J.P. Quetiapine for insomnia: A review of the literature. *Am. J. Health Syst. Pharm.* **2014**, *71*, 394–402. [CrossRef]
7. Kreys, T.J.; Phan, S.V. A literature review of quetiapine for generalized anxiety disorder. *Pharmacotherapy* **2015**, *35*, 175–188. [CrossRef]
8. Sacks, O. *Musicophilia-La Musique, le Cerveau et Nous*; Média Diffusion: Paris, France, 2018.
9. Kalari, V.K.; Morrison, P.E.; Budman, C.L. Atypical antipsychotics for treatment of Tourette syndrome. In *International Review of Movement Disorders*; Elsevier: Amsterdam, The Netherlands, 2022; Volume 4, pp. 203–235.
10. Fischer, B.A.; Boggs, D.L. The role of antihistaminic effects in the misuse of quetiapine: A case report and review of the literature. *Neurosci. Biobehav. Rev.* **2010**, *34*, 555–558. [CrossRef]
11. Terry, N.; Margolis, K.G. Serotonergic Mechanisms Regulating the GI Tract: Experimental Evidence and Therapeutic Relevance. *Handb. Exp. Pharmacol.* **2017**, *239*, 319–342. [CrossRef]
12. Moreines, J.L.; Owrutsky, Z.L.; Gagnon, K.G.; Grace, A.A. Divergent effects of acute and repeated quetiapine treatment on dopamine neuron activity in normal vs. chronic mild stress induced hypodopaminergic states. *Transl. Psychiatry* **2017**, *7*, 1275. [CrossRef]
13. Barandouzi, Z.A.; Lee, J.; Del Carmen Rosas, M.; Chen, J.; Henderson, W.A.; Starkweather, A.R.; Cong, X.S. Associations of neurotransmitters and the gut microbiome with emotional distress in mixed type of irritable bowel syndrome. *Sci. Rep.* **2022**, *12*, 1648. [CrossRef]
14. Mlambo, R.; Liu, J.; Wang, Q.; Tan, S.; Chen, C. Receptors Involved in Mental Disorders and the Use of Clozapine, Chlorpromazine, Olanzapine, and Aripiprazole to Treat Mental Disorders. *Pharmaceuticals* **2023**, *16*, 603. [CrossRef]
15. DeVane, C.L.; Nemeroff, C.B. Clinical pharmacokinetics of quetiapine: An atypical antipsychotic. *Clin. Pharmacokinet.* **2001**, *40*, 509–522. [CrossRef]

16. Pilgrim, J.L.; Drummer, O.H. The toxicology and comorbidities of fatal cases involving quetiapine. *Forensic Sci. Med. Pathol.* **2013**, *9*, 170–176. [CrossRef]
17. Gibiino, S.; Trappoli, A.; Balzarro, B.; Atti, A.R.; De Ronchi, D. Coma After Quetiapine Fumarate Intentional Overdose in a 71-year-old Man: A Case Report. *Drug Saf. Case Rep.* **2015**, *2*, 3. [CrossRef]
18. Parker, D.R.; McIntyre, I.M. Case studies of postmortem quetiapine: Therapeutic or toxic concentrations? *J. Anal. Toxicol.* **2005**, *29*, 407–412. [CrossRef]
19. Andersen, F.D.; Simonsen, U.; Andersen, C.U. Quetiapine and other antipsychotics combined with opioids in legal autopsy cases: A random finding or cause of fatal outcome? *Basic Clin. Pharmacol. Toxicol.* **2021**, *128*, 66–79. [CrossRef]
20. Wu, C.S.; Tsai, Y.T.; Tsai, H.J. Antipsychotic drugs and the risk of ventricular arrhythmia and/or sudden cardiac death: A nation-wide case-crossover study. *J. Am. Heart Assoc.* **2015**, *4*, e001568. [CrossRef]
21. Saito, T.; Tsuji, T.; Namera, A.; Morita, S.; Nakagawa, Y. Comparison of serum and whole blood concentrations in quetiapine overdose cases. *Forensic Toxicol.* **2022**, *40*, 403–406. [CrossRef]
22. Ostad Haji, E.; Wagner, S.; Fric, M.; Laux, G.; Pittermann, P.; Roschke, J.; Hiemke, C. Quetiapine and norquetiapine serum concentrations and clinical effects in depressed patients under augmentation therapy with quetiapine. *Ther. Drug Monit.* **2013**, *35*, 539–545. [CrossRef]
23. Balit, C.R.; Isbister, G.K.; Hackett, L.P.; Whyte, I.M. Quetiapine poisoning: A case series. *Ann. Emerg. Med.* **2003**, *42*, 751–758. [CrossRef]
24. Cubeddu, L.X. Iatrogenic QT Abnormalities and Fatal Arrhythmias: Mechanisms and Clinical Significance. *Curr. Cardiol. Rev.* **2009**, *5*, 166–176. [CrossRef]
25. El Mazloum, R.; Snenghi, R.; Zorzi, A.; Zilio, F.; Dorigo, A.; Montisci, R.; Corrado, D.; Montisci, M. Out-of-hospital cardiac arrest after acute cocaine intoxication associated with Brugada ECG patterns: Insights into physiopathologic mechanisms and implications for therapy. *Int. J. Cardiol.* **2015**, *195*, 245–249. [CrossRef] [PubMed]
26. Montisci, M.; Thiene, G.; Ferrara, S.D.; Basso, C. Cannabis and cocaine: A lethal cocktail triggering coronary sudden death. *Cardiovasc. Pathol.* **2008**, *17*, 344–346. [CrossRef] [PubMed]
27. Andersen, F.D.; Joca, S.; Hvingelby, V.; Arjmand, S.; Pinilla, E.; Steffensen, S.C.; Simonsen, U.; Andersen, C.U. Combined effects of quetiapine and opioids: A study of autopsy cases, drug users and sedation in rats. *Addict. Biol.* **2022**, *27*, e13214. [CrossRef] [PubMed]
28. Khokhar, M.A.; Rathbone, J. Droperidol for psychosis-induced aggression or agitation. *Cochrane Database Syst. Rev.* **2016**, *12*, CD002830. [CrossRef] [PubMed]
29. Culebras, X.; Corpataux, J.B.; Gaggero, G.; Tramer, M.R. The antiemetic efficacy of droperidol added to morphine patient-controlled analgesia: A randomized, controlled, multicenter dose-finding study. *Anesth. Analg.* **2003**, *97*, 816–821. [CrossRef] [PubMed]
30. Zargar, S.; Wani, T.A.; Alsaif, N.A.; Khayyat, A.I.A. A Comprehensive Investigation of Interactions between Antipsychotic Drug Quetiapine and Human Serum Albumin Using Multi-Spectroscopic, Biochemical, and Molecular Modeling Approaches. *Molecules* **2022**, *27*, 2589. [CrossRef] [PubMed]
31. Narala, A.; Veerabrahma, K. Preparation, Characterization and Evaluation of Quetiapine Fumarate Solid Lipid Nanoparticles to Improve the Oral Bioavailability. *J. Pharm.* **2013**, *2013*, 265741. [CrossRef]
32. Junior, E.; Duarte, L.; Suenaga, E.; de Carvalho Cruz, A.; Nakaie, C. Comparative bioavailability of two quetiapine formulations in healthy volunteers after a single dose administration. *J. Bioequiv Availab.* **2011**, *3*, 178–181. [CrossRef]
33. Schonborn, J.L.; Gwinnutt, C. The Role of the Liver in Drug Metabolism Anaesthesia Tutorial of the Week 179 17th May 2010. *ATOTW* **2010**. Available online: https://resources.wfsahq.org/atotw/the-role-of-the-liver-in-drug-metabolism/ (accessed on 20 November 2023).
34. Waal, H.; Vold, J.H.; Skurtveit, S.O. Quetiapine abuse—Myth or reality? *Tidsskr. Nor. Laegeforen* **2020**, *140*, 1228–1230. [CrossRef]
35. Ybanez, L.; Spiller, H.A.; Badeti, J.; Casavant, M.J.; Rine, N.; Michaels, N.L.; Zhu, M.; Smith, G.A. Suspected suicides and suicide attempts involving antipsychotic or sedative-hypnotic medications reported to America's Poison Centers, 2000–2021. *Clin. Toxicol.* **2023**, *61*, 294–304. [CrossRef] [PubMed]
36. Cetin, N.; Konuk, N. Suicide attempt with a very high dose of quetiapine. *Klin. Psikofarmakol. Bul.-Bull. Clin. Psychopharmacol.* **2011**, *21*, 67–69. [CrossRef]
37. Kinoshita, H.; Tanaka, N.; Kumihashi, M.; Jamal, G.; Ito, A.; Yamashita, T.; Ozawa, Y.; Ameno, K. An autopsy case of drowning under the influence of multiple psychotropic drugs. *Arch. Med. Sadowej Kryminol.* **2019**, *69*, 222–227. [CrossRef]
38. Burke, M.P.; Path, D.F.; Alamad, S.; Dip, G.; Opeskin, K. Death by smothering following forced quetiapine administration in an infant. *Am. J. Forensic Med. Pathol.* **2004**, *25*, 243–245. [CrossRef] [PubMed]
39. Bertol, E.; Vaiano, F.; Argo, A.; Zerbo, S.; Trignano, C.; Protani, S.; Favretto, D. Overdose of Quetiapine-A Case Report with QT Prolongation. *Toxics* **2021**, *9*, 339. [CrossRef] [PubMed]
40. Office for National Statistics (UK). Number of Drug-Related Deaths Due to Quetiapine Use in England and Wales from 1998 to 2021. Available online: https://www.ons.gov.uk/file?uri=/peoplepopulationandcommunity/birthsdeathsandmarriages/deaths/datasets/deathsrelatedtodrugpoisoningbyselectedsubstances/2019registrations/2019pivot3.xlsx (accessed on 25 October 2023).
41. Lee, J.; Pilgrim, J.; Gerostamoulos, D.; Robinson, J.; Wong, A. Increasing rates of quetiapine overdose, misuse, and mortality in Victoria, Australia. *Drug Alcohol. Depend.* **2018**, *187*, 95–99. [CrossRef]

42. Kales, H.C.; Kim, H.M.; Zivin, K.; Valenstein, M.; Seyfried, L.S.; Chiang, C.; Cunningham, F.; Schneider, L.S.; Blow, F.C. Risk of mortality among individual antipsychotics in patients with dementia. *Am. J. Psychiatry* **2012**, *169*, 71–79. [CrossRef]
43. Maust, D.T.; Kim, H.M.; Seyfried, L.S.; Chiang, C.; Kavanagh, J.; Schneider, L.S.; Kales, H.C. Antipsychotics, other psychotropics, and the risk of death in patients with dementia: Number needed to harm. *JAMA Psychiatry* **2015**, *72*, 438–445. [CrossRef]
44. Breivik, H.; Frost, J.; Lokken, T.N.; Slordal, L. Post mortem tissue distribution of quetiapine in forensic autopsies. *Forensic Sci. Int.* **2020**, *315*, 110413. [CrossRef]
45. Vignali, C.; Freni, F.; Magnani, C.; Moretti, M.; Siodambro, C.; Groppi, A.; Osculati, A.M.M.; Morini, L. Distribution of quetiapine and metabolites in biological fluids and tissues. *Forensic Sci. Int.* **2020**, *307*, 110108. [CrossRef]
46. Aly, S.M.; Gish, A.; Hakim, F.; Guelmi, D.; Mesli, V.; Hédouin, V.; Allorge, D.; Gaulier, J.M. In the case of extensively putrefied bodies, the analysis of entomological samples may support and complement the toxicological results obtained with other alternative matrices. *Leg. Med.* **2023**, *63*, 102261. [CrossRef] [PubMed]
47. Nishio, T.; Toukairin, Y.; Hoshi, T.; Arai, T.; Nogami, M. Quantification of nine psychotropic drugs in postmortem dried blood spot samples by liquid chromatography-tandem mass spectrometry for simple toxicological analysis. *J. Pharm. Biomed. Anal.* **2023**, *233*, 115438. [CrossRef]
48. Tawfik, G.M.; Dila, K.A.S.; Mohamed, M.Y.F.; Tam, D.N.H.; Kien, N.D.; Ahmed, A.M.; Huy, N.T. A step by step guide for conducting a systematic review and meta-analysis with simulation data. *Trop. Med. Health* **2019**, *47*, 46. [CrossRef] [PubMed]
49. Page, M.J.; McKenzie, J.E.; Bossuyt, P.M.; Boutron, I.; Hoffmann, T.C.; Mulrow, C.D.; Shamseer, L.; Tetzlaff, J.M.; Akl, E.A.; Brennan, S.E.; et al. The PRISMA 2020 statement: An updated guideline for reporting systematic reviews. *Syst. Rev.* **2021**, *10*, 89. [CrossRef] [PubMed]
50. Anderson, D.T.; Fritz, K.L. Quetiapine (Seroquel) concentrations in seven postmortem cases. *J. Anal. Toxicol.* **2000**, *24*, 300–304. [CrossRef] [PubMed]
51. Hopenwasser, J.; Mozayani, A.; Danielson, T.J.; Harbin, J.; Narula, H.S.; Posey, D.H.; Shrode, P.W.; Wilson, S.K.; Li, R.; Sanchez, L.A. Postmortem distribution of the novel antipsychotic drug quetiapine. *J. Anal. Toxicol.* **2004**, *28*, 264–267. [CrossRef]
52. Vaja, R.; Rana, M. Drugs and the liver. *Anaesth. Intensive Care Med.* **2020**, *21*, 517–523. [CrossRef]
53. Jones, G.R.; Singer, P.P. Drugs-of-Abuse in Liver. *Drug Test. Altern. Biol. Specim.* **2008**, 139–156. [CrossRef]
54. Fuke, C.; Berry, C.L.; Pounder, D.J. Postmortem diffusion of ingested and aspirated paint thinner. *Forensic Sci. Int.* **1996**, *78*, 199–207. [CrossRef]
55. Pounder, D.J.; Davies, J.I. Zopiclone poisoning: Tissue distribution and potential for postmortem diffusion. *Forensic Sci. Int.* **1994**, *65*, 177–183. [CrossRef]
56. LiverTox, L. *Clinical and Research Information on Drug-Induced Liver Injury [Internet] Bethesda*; National Institute of Diabetes and Digestive and Kidney Diseases: Bethesda, MD, USA, 2012.
57. Abdel-Misih, S.R.; Bloomston, M. Liver anatomy. *Surg. Clin. N. Am.* **2010**, *90*, 643–653. [CrossRef] [PubMed]
58. Aguiar, J.A.; Riaz, A.; Thornburg, B. Biliary Anatomy. *Semin. Interv. Radiol.* **2021**, *38*, 251–254. [CrossRef] [PubMed]
59. Hamsa, A.; Karumandampalayam Shanmugaramasamy, K.; Kariyarambath, P.; Kathirvel, S. Quetiapine Fumarate: A Review of Analytical Methods. *J. Chromatogr. Sci.* **2022**, *61*, bmac100. [CrossRef] [PubMed]
60. Liu, T.L.; Fang, L.S.; Liou, J.R.; Dai, J.S.; Chen, Y.L. Determination of quetiapine and its metabolites in plasma by field-enhanced sample stacking. *J. Food Drug Anal.* **2021**, *29*, 709–716. [CrossRef] [PubMed]
61. Lee, H.J.; Choi, J.S.; Choi, B.H.; Hahn, S.J. Effects of norquetiapine, the active metabolite of quetiapine, on cloned hERG potassium channels. *Neurosci. Lett.* **2018**, *664*, 66–73. [CrossRef] [PubMed]
62. Ortega-Ruiz, M.; Soria-Chacartegui, P.; Villapalos-García, G.; Abad-Santos, F.; Zubiaur, P. The Pharmacogenetics of Treatment with Quetiapine. *Future Pharmacol.* **2022**, *2*, 276–286. [CrossRef]
63. Muller, C.; Reuter, H.; Dohmen, C. Intoxication after extreme oral overdose of quetiapine to attempt suicide: Pharmacological concerns of side effects. *Case Rep. Med.* **2009**, *2009*, 371698. [CrossRef] [PubMed]
64. Babyak, J.M.; Lee, J.A. Toxicological emergencies. In *BSAVA Manual of Canine and Feline Emergency and Critical Care*; BSAVA Library: Gloucester, UK, 2018; pp. 304–317.
65. Kartasheva-Ebertz, D.; Gaston, J.; Lair-Mehiri, L.; Massault, P.P.; Scatton, O.; Vaillant, J.C.; Morozov, V.A.; Pol, S.; Lagaye, S. Adult human liver slice cultures: Modelling of liver fibrosis and evaluation of new anti-fibrotic drugs. *World J. Hepatol.* **2021**, *13*, 187–217. [CrossRef]
66. Saxton, S.H.; Stevens, K.R. 2D and 3D liver models. *J. Hepatol.* **2023**, *78*, 873–875. [CrossRef]
67. Hernández-Mesa, M.; Moreno-González, D. Current Role of Mass Spectrometry in the Determination of Pesticide Residues in Food. *Separations* **2022**, *9*, 148. [CrossRef]
68. Poloznikov, A.; Gazaryan, I.; Shkurnikov, M.; Nikulin, S.; Drapkina, O.; Baranova, A.; Tonevitsky, A. In vitro and in silico liver models: Current trends, challenges and opportunities. *ALTEX* **2018**, *35*, 397–412. [CrossRef] [PubMed]
69. Yang, H.; Sun, L.; Pang, Y.; Hu, D.; Xu, H.; Mao, S.; Peng, W.; Wang, Y.; Xu, Y.; Zheng, Y.C.; et al. Three-dimensional bioprinted hepatorganoids prolong survival of mice with liver failure. *Gut* **2021**, *70*, 567–574. [CrossRef] [PubMed]
70. Fischer, I.; Milton, C.; Wallace, H. Toxicity testing is evolving! *Toxicol. Res.* **2020**, *9*, 67–80. [CrossRef] [PubMed]

71. Abstracts of the10th International ISSX meeting, September 29-October 3, 2013, Toronto, Ontario, Canada. *Drug Metab. Rev.* **2014**, *45* (Suppl. S1), 1–286. [CrossRef]
72. Le Dare, B.; Ferron, P.J.; Allard, P.M.; Clement, B.; Morel, I.; Gicquel, T. New insights into quetiapine metabolism using molecular networking. *Sci. Rep.* **2020**, *10*, 19921. [CrossRef] [PubMed]
73. Carvalho Henriques, B.; Yang, E.H.; Lapetina, D.; Carr, M.S.; Yavorskyy, V.; Hague, J.; Aitchison, K.J. How Can Drug Metabolism and Transporter Genetics Inform Psychotropic Prescribing? *Front. Genet.* **2020**, *11*, 491895. [CrossRef] [PubMed]
74. Okumura, A.; Tanimizu, N. Preparation of Functional Human Hepatocytes Ex Vivo. *Methods Mol. Biol.* **2022**, *2544*, 269–278. [CrossRef] [PubMed]
75. Frances, D.; Ronco, M.T.; Ochoa, E.; Alvarez, M.L.; Quiroga, A.; Parody, J.P.; Monti, J.; Carrillo, M.C.; Carnovale, C.E. Oxidative stress in primary culture hepatocytes isolated from partially hepatectomized rats. *Can. J. Physiol. Pharmacol.* **2007**, *85*, 1047–1051. [CrossRef]
76. Rodrigues, R.M.; Heymans, A.; De Boe, V.; Sachinidis, A.; Chaudhari, U.; Govaere, O.; Roskams, T.; Vanhaecke, T.; Rogiers, V.; De Kock, J. Toxicogenomics-based prediction of acetaminophen-induced liver injury using human hepatic cell systems. *Toxicol. Lett.* **2016**, *240*, 50–59. [CrossRef]
77. De Siervi, S.; Turato, C. Liver Organoids as an In Vitro Model to Study Primary Liver Cancer. *Int. J. Mol. Sci.* **2023**, *24*, 4529. [CrossRef]
78. Lee, J.H.; Ho, K.L.; Fan, S.K. Liver microsystems in vitro for drug response. *J. Biomed. Sci.* **2019**, *26*, 88. [CrossRef] [PubMed]
79. Dede, E.; Tindall, M.J.; Cherrie, J.W.; Hankin, S.; Collins, C. Physiologically-based pharmacokinetic and toxicokinetic models for estimating human exposure to five toxic elements through oral ingestion. *Environ. Toxicol. Pharmacol.* **2018**, *57*, 104–114. [CrossRef] [PubMed]
80. Bravo-Gomez, M.E.; Camacho-Garcia, L.N.; Castillo-Alanis, L.A.; Mendoza-Melendez, M.A.; Quijano-Mateos, A. Revisiting a physiologically based pharmacokinetic model for cocaine with a forensic scope. *Toxicol. Res.* **2019**, *8*, 432–446. [CrossRef] [PubMed]
81. Adachi, K.; Beppu, S.; Nishiyama, K.; Shimizu, M.; Yamazaki, H. Pharmacokinetics of duloxetine self-administered in overdose with quetiapine and other antipsychotic drugs in a Japanese patient admitted to hospital. *J. Pharm. Health Care Sci.* **2021**, *7*, 6. [CrossRef] [PubMed]
82. Sager, J.E.; Yu, J.; Ragueneau-Majlessi, I.; Isoherranen, N. Physiologically Based Pharmacokinetic (PBPK) Modeling and Simulation Approaches: A Systematic Review of Published Models, Applications, and Model Verification. *Drug Metab. Dispos.* **2015**, *43*, 1823–1837. [CrossRef] [PubMed]
83. Mamada, H.; Iwamoto, K.; Nomura, Y.; Uesawa, Y. Predicting blood-to-plasma concentration ratios of drugs from chemical structures and volumes of distribution in humans. *Mol. Divers.* **2021**, *25*, 1261–1270. [CrossRef] [PubMed]
84. Deng, J.; Wei, W.; Chen, Z.; Lin, B.; Zhao, W.; Luo, Y.; Zhang, X. Engineered Liver-on-a-Chip Platform to Mimic Liver Functions and Its Biomedical Applications: A Review. *Micromachines* **2019**, *10*, 676. [CrossRef]
85. Mirzazadeh, M.; Shine, B. Evidence Based Pathology and Laboratory Medicine. *Ann. Clin. Biochem.* **2012**, 49. [CrossRef]
86. Jones, A.W.; Holmgren, A.; Ahlner, J. Post-mortem concentrations of drugs determined in femoral blood in single-drug fatalities compared with multi-drug poisoning deaths. *Forensic Sci. Int.* **2016**, *267*, 96–103. [CrossRef]
87. Skov, L.; Johansen, S.S.; Linnet, K. Postmortem Quetiapine Reference Concentrations in Brain and Blood. *J. Anal. Toxicol.* **2015**, *39*, 557–561. [CrossRef]
88. Burghardt, K.J.; Ward, K.M.; Sanders, E.J.; Howlett, B.H.; Seyoum, B.; Yi, Z. Atypical Antipsychotics and the Human Skeletal Muscle Lipidome. *Metabolites* **2018**, *8*, 64. [CrossRef] [PubMed]
89. Breivik, H.; Lokken, T.N.; Slordal, L.; Frost, J. A Validated Method for the Simultaneous Determination of Quetiapine, Clozapine and Mirtazapine in Postmortem Blood and Tissue Samples. *J. Anal. Toxicol.* **2020**, *44*, 440–448. [CrossRef] [PubMed]
90. de Campos, E.G.; da Costa, B.R.B.; Dos Santos, F.S.; Monedeiro, F.; Alves, M.N.R.; Santos Junior, W.J.R.; De Martinis, B.S. Alternative matrices in forensic toxicology: A critical review. *Forensic Toxicol.* **2022**, *40*, 1–18. [CrossRef] [PubMed]
91. Favretto, D.; Stocchero, G.; Nalesso, A.; Vogliardi, S.; Boscolo-Berto, R.; Montisci, M.; Ferrara, S.D. Monitoring haloperidol exposure in body fluids and hair of children by liquid chromatography-high-resolution mass spectrometry. *Ther. Drug Monit.* **2013**, *35*, 493–501. [CrossRef] [PubMed]
92. Gunther, K.N.; Johansen, S.S.; Nielsen, M.K.K.; Wicktor, P.; Banner, J.; Linnet, K. Post-mortem quetiapine concentrations in hair segments of psychiatric patients—Correlation between hair concentration, dose and concentration in blood. *Forensic Sci. Int.* **2018**, *285*, 58–64. [CrossRef] [PubMed]
93. Yang, H.; Liu, C.; Zhu, C.; Zheng, Y.; Li, J.; Zhu, Q.; Wang, H.; Fang, X.; Liu, Q.; Liang, M.; et al. Determination of ten antipsychotics in blood, hair and nails: Validation of a LC-MS/MS method and forensic application of keratinized matrix analysis. *J. Pharm. Biomed. Anal.* **2023**, *234*, 115557. [CrossRef]
94. Ferrara, S.D.; Cecchetto, G.; Cecchi, R.; Favretto, D.; Grabherr, S.; Ishikawa, T.; Kondo, T.; Montisci, M.; Pfeiffer, H.; Bonati, M.R.; et al. Back to the Future—Part 2. Post-mortem assessment and evolutionary role of the bio-medicolegal sciences. *Int. J. Leg. Med.* **2017**, *131*, 1085–1101. [CrossRef]

95. Krumbiegel, F.; Hastedt, M.; Westendorf, L.; Niebel, A.; Methling, M.; Parr, M.K.; Tsokos, M. The use of nails as an alternative matrix for the long-term detection of previous drug intake: Validation of sensitive UHPLC-MS/MS methods for the quantification of 76 substances and comparison of analytical results for drugs in nail and hair samples. *Forensic Sci. Med. Pathol.* **2016**, *12*, 416–434. [CrossRef]
96. Cobo-Golpe, M.; de-Castro-Ríos, A.; Cruz, A.; Páramo, M.; López-Rivadulla, M.; Lendoiro, E. Determination of antipsychotic drugs in nails and hair by liquid chromatography tandem mass spectrometry and evaluation of their incorporation into keratinized matrices. *J. Pharm. Biomed. Anal.* **2020**, *189*, 113443. [CrossRef]

Disclaimer/Publisher's Note: The statements, opinions and data contained in all publications are solely those of the individual author(s) and contributor(s) and not of MDPI and/or the editor(s). MDPI and/or the editor(s) disclaim responsibility for any injury to people or property resulting from any ideas, methods, instructions or products referred to in the content.

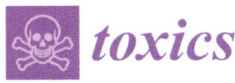

Article

11-Nor-9-Carboxy Tetrahydrocannabinol Distribution in Fluid from the Chest Cavity in Cannabis-Related Post-Mortem Cases

Torki A. Zughaibi [1,2,*], Hassan Alharbi [3], Adel Al-Saadi [3], Abdulnasser E. Alzahrani [3] and Ahmed I. Al-Asmari [4,*]

1. Department of Medical Laboratory Sciences, Faculty of Applied Medical Sciences, King Abdulaziz University, Jeddah 21589, Saudi Arabia
2. King Fahd Medical Research Center, King Abdulaziz University, Jeddah 21589, Saudi Arabia
3. Poison Control and Forensic Chemistry Center, Ministry of Health, Jeddah 21176, Saudi Arabia
4. Special Toxicological Analysis Unit, Pathology and Laboratory Medicine DPLM, King Faisal Specialist Hospital and Research Center, P.O. Box 3354, Riyadh 11211, Saudi Arabia
* Correspondence: taalzughaibi@kau.edu.sa (T.A.Z.); ahmadalasmari@yahoo.com (A.I.A.-A.)

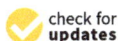

Citation: Zughaibi, T.A.; Alharbi, H.; Al-Saadi, A.; Alzahrani, A.E.; Al-Asmari, A.I. 11-Nor-9-Carboxy Tetrahydrocannabinol Distribution in Fluid from the Chest Cavity in Cannabis-Related Post-Mortem Cases. *Toxics* 2023, *11*, 740. https://doi.org/10.3390/toxics11090740

Academic Editor: Eric J. F. Franssen

Received: 4 July 2023
Revised: 8 August 2023
Accepted: 25 August 2023
Published: 29 August 2023

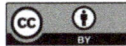

Copyright: © 2023 by the authors. Licensee MDPI, Basel, Switzerland. This article is an open access article distributed under the terms and conditions of the Creative Commons Attribution (CC BY) license (https:// creativecommons.org/licenses/by/ 4.0/).

Abstract: In this study, the presence of 11-nor-Δ^9-carboxy tetrahydrocannabinol (THC-COOH) in postmortem fluid obtained from the chest cavity (FCC) of postmortem cases collected from drug-related fatalities or criminal-related deaths in Jeddah, Saudi Arabia, was investigated to evaluate its suitability for use as a complementary specimen to blood and biological specimens in cases where no bodily fluids are available or suitable for analysis. The relationships between THC-COOH concentrations in the FCC samples and age, body mass index (BMI), polydrug intoxication, manner, and cause of death were investigated. Methods: Fifteen postmortem cases of FCC were analyzed using fully validated liquid chromatography-positive-electrospray ionization tandem mass spectrometry (LC-MS/MS). Results: FCC samples were collected from 15 postmortem cases; only THC-COOH tested positive, with a median concentration of 480 ng/mL (range = 80–3010 ng/mL). THC-COOH in FCC were higher than THC-COOH in all tested specimens with exception to bile, the median ratio FCC/blood with sodium fluoride, FCC/urine, FCC/gastric content, FCC/bile, FCC/liver, FCC/kidney, FCC/brain, FCC/stomach wall, FCC/lung, and FCC/intestine tissue were 48, 2, 0.2, 6, 4, 6, 102, 11, 5 and 10-fold, respectively. Conclusion: This is the first postmortem report of THC-COOH in the FCC using cannabinoid-related analysis. The FCC samples were liquid, easy to manipulate, and extracted using the same procedure as the blood samples. The source of THC-COOH detected in FCC could be derived from the surrounding organs due to postmortem redistribution or contamination due to postmortem changes after death. THC-COOH, which is stored in adipose tissues, could be a major source of THC-COOH found in the FCC.

Keywords: 11-nor-Δ^9-carboxy tetrahydrocannabinol; post-mortem analysis; fluid; chest cavity; LC-MS/MS

1. Introduction

Cannabis is an increasingly harmful product that is used worldwide [1]. The American National Survey on Drug Use and Health reported that 16% of the American population (43.5 million) used marijuana in 2018 [2,3]. In Canada, 3.8% of drivers were found positive for cannabis, which is reported to increase the risk of automobile accidents two-fold [4]. Cannabis is considered a substance of abuse in the Middle East and North Africa (MENA). In Arab nations, apart from Lebanon, cannabis is considered as a substance of abuse [5]. However, rarely has the reporting on the role of cannabis use in MENA investigated antemortem of postmortem cases. Indirectly, cannabis is commonly detected in postmortem cases with powerful drugs of abuse such as heroin and methamphetamine [6,7]. The impact of cannabis in the cause of death is not fully understood, and it is a paramount task for forensic toxicologists to provide information regarding its role in these deaths;

therefore, forensic postmortem investigations are required. Consequently, identification of cannabinoids and their metabolites is crucial for forensic toxicologists [8,9].

In human cadavers, the active compound of cannabis (Δ^9-tetrahydrocannabinol (THC)) metabolism is well known, and this compound has a psychoactive effect following cannabis administration [10]. THC is converted to 11-hydroxy-tetrahydrocannabinol (THC-OH) and then metabolized to 11-nor-Δ^9-carboxy tetrahydrocannabinol (THC-COOH) [11]. Until recently, the inclusion of THC and its metabolites in postmortem analysis has gained less interest due to the common belief that it does not contribute to the cause of death. Numerous measurement methods have been reported for the analysis of these metabolites in ante-mortem specimens, particularly for drivers under the influence of drugs and workplace drug testing. Most of these challenges are encountered due to the low THC and THC-OH concentrations in the blood, and most of the THC and its metabolites are converted to more polar metabolites by glucuronidation. Free THC and its metabolites were rarely detected in urine samples. The hydrolysis step becomes a cornerstone for the detection of THC and its major metabolite, THC-COOH, in bodily and tissue specimens, regardless of the techniques used for analysis. Therefore, two challenges must be considered when developing methods for THC and metabolite analyses. First, the low concentration of active THC metabolites in the specimens of interest requires sensitive analytical techniques. Second, the samples were prepared to be suitable for testing the free analytes of interest without preliminary sample preparation for analyzing the polar conjugated metabolites of these analytes. The approach of testing glucuronide metabolites has received little attention in previous postmortem analyses for two main reasons. The first is that not all glucuronide metabolites and their internal standards are commercially available. The second reason is that testing glucuronide metabolites using gas chromatography-mass spectrometry (GC-MS) is not appropriate and is time consuming because of these polar metabolites. In postmortem testing for cannabinoids, more than one procedure is often used to obtain free THC and its metabolites in non-blood specimens; for example, a combination of protein precipitation, following by alkaline or enzymatic hydrolysis, and then subjected to either liquid-liquid extraction (LE) or solid phase extraction (SPE), followed by derivatization using GC-MS. The use of LC-MS techniques has a great impact on the postmortem testing of cannabinoids, and several advantages can be gained when using LC-MS techniques over GC-MS, such as the lack of derivatizing agents required [12,13], in cases where urine samples, direct analysis without sample pretreatment approach into LC-MS, and the most important cannabinoid glucuronide can be directly measured without hydrolysis steps [8,14].

THC and THC-COOH have been the most frequently detected cannabis metabolites in previous studies, and few studies have reported THC-OH [8,9,11,14,15]. It is well known that the distribution of parent drugs and their metabolites varies among individuals due to their tolerance, occurrence of usage, presence of other drug(s), state of health of study subjects, stability of the target analytes in antemortem and postmortem cases, and during storage in test tubes. One of the goals of testing parents and metabolites is to understand the time of intake; however, this has been poorly reported in previous studies. In fact, each cannabinoid metabolite is unique and time-dependent. THC and THC-OH appear shortly following cannabis demonstration, which is similar to THC-COOH; however, the latter could be determined in human specimens for a longer time, even without THC and THC. THC-COOH is stored in fatty adipose tissues, continues to leach into the blood circulation, and is finally excreted with urine, which makes detection of THC-COOH unsuitable for distinguishing the time of use. The appearance of THC and THC-OH in the blood has been suggested as a tool to estimate the state of impairment and recent cannabinoids used [9,11].

Blood is the sample of choice in most forensic applications, particularly postmortem analysis. A history of drug use can be evaluated using urine samples in parallel with blood tests. However, these two distinct specimens may not be available on many postmortem occasions such as traffic accidents and urination before death. Therefore, alternative specimens may be used to obtain data to support cases in hand [2,11,16]. Analysis of these alternative specimens may introduce new challenges regarding the homogeneous nature of these specimens, that is, tissue specimens (skeletal muscle, liver, gallbladder, kidneys, spleen, and brain tissues).

In situations where blood or other bodily fluids are unattainable during autopsy examination, it is crucial to explore dependable non-blood postmortem samples as alternative or complementary sources for quantifying and identifying THC and its metabolites. None of the body fluids were deemed appropriate for cases that were received at the JPCC. Alternative samples, such as liver, kidneys, stomach wall, and brain, were collected. In some cases, the fluid from the chest cavity (FCC), specifically from the pleural cavity, was sent for analysis.

Notably, high concentrations of THC-COOH were obtained when the FCC was tested for cannabinoids; this is novel, and no information regarding FCC testing is available in the literature. Thus, FCC from other cannabinoid-positive cases that conceded positive results for THC or its metabolites were further evaluated to investigate the concentration of THC-COOH in the FCC.

To the best of the authors' knowledge, this is the first postmortem report of THC-COOH in the FCC. The impact of this approach is to provide suitable and homogenous specimens appropriate for testing analytes of interest that can be extracted easily, when compared to sold tissues specimens, which are always tested in such cases where no blood is available. It was investigated if these analytes' concentrations differ from bodily fluids and tissue specimen's concentration and which analytes are mostly detected in FCC. The purpose of this study was to study the value of non-blood specimens including, for the first time, FCC. In addition, these results were compared with other postmortem specimen results from previously published reports.

2. Materials and Methods

2.1. Speciemns Selection

The demography of the deceased in this report (history, sex, age, body mass index (BMI), interval time (PMI), and mode of death) was acquired from the Forensic Postmortem Jeddah database (FTRJ), which is an online database for medicolegal cases received by the Jeddah Toxicology Centre (JTC), Jeddah, Saudi Arabia.

2.2. Specimens Collection

In this investigation, the same protocol used for sample collection in our previous cannabinoid investigations was followed [9,15,17]. Briefly, blood was collected in sample tubes containing at least 1–2% sodium fluoride (BNaF). All BNaF was drawn from subclavian vein, while the liver was collected from at least three different sites throughout the deep right lobe of the liver in order to avoid contamination. Kidney tissues were taken from both the right and left kidneys, at the center of each kidney. Urine samples were collected from the bladder tissue using a clean syringe. Gastric contents obtained at autopsy were collected and used for analysis. Bile in liquid form was collected when it was possible. The stomach wall (W-Stomach), lung, brain, and small intestine (S. intestine) tissue were collected from 3–5 sites of these tissues.

2.3. Bodily and Tissues Sample Preparation

2.3.1. Non-Hydrolyzed Specimens

One mL of BNaF and FCC were kept separately in 15 mL sample glass tubes (screw-capped). Next, 50 µL of internal standards containing THC-OH-d_3, THC-COOH-d_9, and THC-d_3 (50 ng/mL) were transferred to each calibration and test sample and mixed thoroughly.

2.3.2. Hydrolyzed Specimens

In this study, one milliliter of urine, bile, and gastric content were subjected to alkaline hydrolysis. Then, 50 µL of internal standards containing THC-OH-d_3, THC-COOH-d_9, and THC-d$_3$ (50 ng/mL) were transferred to each calibration and test sample and mixed thoroughly. Sodium hydroxide (NaOH) (10 N) was added to each specimen (200 µL). All the urine, bile, and gastric content samples were placed in a water bath at 60 °C for at least 20 min to facilitate hydrolysis. The pH of the samples was adjusted to 3.5, using 2 mL of concentrated glacial acetic acid (GAA), and placed in a cold place for at least 5 min. For the brain, S-Intestine, W-Stomach, and Lung tissues, a gram of each tissue was weighed and then diluted using aqueous 1% sodium fluoride. Tissue at a ratio of 2:1 was added into a stomacher bag and homogenized for 5 min in a Stomacher machine (Seward Limited, Worthing, UK). Homogenized tissue (500 mg) was transferred to a new test tube. Then, 50 µL of the same internal standard was spiked into each tube. Next, 200 µL of NaOH (10 N) was transferred to each test tube, which was placed in a water bath at 60 °C for at least 20 min to facilitate hydrolysis. After cooling the sample tubes for 5 min, the sample pH was adjusted to 2 mL of GAA. The specimens were then transferred for centrifugation for 10 min at 2200× g. Finally, the supernatant was transferred into a clean test tube.

2.3.3. Solid Phase Extraction

As detailed in the Al-Asmari report, all samples were processed using labeled Clean Screen® cartridges for extraction [9,15]. Briefly, the SPE system was positioned on a vacuum manifold. Initially, the column was preconditioned by adding first adding 3 mL of methanol, then adding 3 mL of deionized water (H$_2$O-D) to each cartridge, and 1 mL of hydrochloric acid (HCl, 0.1 M). Next, the supernatant of the specimens prepared above was transferred onto labelled SPE cartridges and allowed to pass through the gravity force. Next, the SPE cartridges were washed with 2 mL of H$_2$O-D, followed by the addition of 1 mL of a solution containing HCl (0.1 M) and acetonitrile (70:30). The SPE cartridges were then placed under vacuum at >10 inches Hg for at least 5 min for drying. Hexane (200 µL) was added for further cleaning. After that, analytes of interest were eluted from labeled SPE cartridges by adding a mixture containing 2 mL of ethyl acetate and hexane (50:50) and then final extracts were dried using nitrogen at 40 °C. Finally, residues were mixed using 100 µL of initial percentages of mobile phase (70% methanol:30% ammonium formate solution (10 mM, pH 3.5) and 1 µL of final extract were injected into the LC-MS/MS.

2.4. LC-MS/MS Conditions

A previously fully validated in-house LC-MS/MS procedure to quantify and detect analytes of interest was used in this study [9]. In these reports, a triple quadrupole mass spectrometer analyzer, operated by electrospray ion, was operated using the multiple reaction monitoring positive ion mode (model: Shimadzu LCMS-8050, Kyoto, Japan) in combination with Ultra-High Performance Liquid Chromatography (UPLC, model: Nexera, Shimadzu, Kyoto, Japan). In this procedure, Raptor Biphenyl column (50 × 3.0 mm, 2.7 µm) and its guard column (model: Raptor Biphenyl, 2.7 µm, 5/3.0 mm; Restek, Bellefonte, PA, USA) were chosen for the separation of analytes; the oven column was set at 40 °C. The autosampler was maintained at 4 °C, and the flow rate was 0.3 mL/min throughout the run. The analytes of interest and their corresponding internal standards were achieved using a gradient elution containing two mobile phases: an aqueous modifier containing ammonium (10 mM, pH 3 (A)) and an organic modifier containing 100% methanol (B). The gradient mobile phase was set at 70% B for one the first min of the run, followed by an increase in B to 95% at 5 min. Solution B was maintained at 95% concentration for 3 min. Finally, 70% of the B solution was installed at 9 min and maintained for the last min of the run at 10 min.

The MS/MS setting was in accordance with our published procedure [9], and spray voltage (7000 V) and temperature (40 °C) were applied in this study. The ionized analytes were then carried into the high vacuum of the MS system. In the MRM mode, Q1 targets the m/z values at 315, 331, and 345, with consequent fragmentation of the target ions at 193, 123, 313, 20, 193, and 299 m/z for THC, THC-OH, and THC-COOH, respectively. For the Q3 fragment, daughter ions were chosen for quantitation purposes. The retention time was within 0.05 of the reference standards and the ion ratios were within +20%.

2.5. Method Validation

The experimental procedures were fully validated as described in detail elsewhere [9,15]. Further optimization was conducted to detect trace concentrations (TR) of THC and THC-OH. In a previous study, the lower limit of quantification (LOQ) were as low as 1 ng/mL and 1 ng/g in body and solid tissue postmortem specimens, respectively [9,15,17]. All calibration curves for THC and its metabolites were found to be linear using calibration ranges of 1–1000 ng/mL (BNaF, VH, urine, bile, gastric contents, and FCC) and 1–1000 ng/g (liver, kidney, and brain tissues) for THC-COOH. Linear calibration curves with coefficients of determination greater than 0.999 were obtained. Within-run precision and between-run precision were evaluated for THC and THC-OH using three quality control standards (QCs) of 25, 100, and 750 for bodily and solid tissues. In the current method, the within- and between-run precisions were better than 10%. The accuracy values were assessed using similar quality control as precision studies, which ranged −8% to +8%. The procedure reported by Matuszewski et al. was followed to measure the effect of the matrix and the recoveries of THC and its metabolites using QCs for each analyte [18]. The matrix effect and recoveries were acceptable, ranging from 78.0% to 122% and 79% to 97%, respectively.

As the variation between concentrations is obvious and can be dependent on health status, chronic use, weight, and other factors, dilution studies should be conducted to ensure that the method is capable of accurately detecting the analytes of interest, as dilution of specimens is also part of the method of extraction and sample preparation. The QCs samples were diluted 100 and 10 times their target concentrations and measured using the described method. All the obtained results were determined and found to be acceptable compared to their target concentrations (±15%). Method selectivity was examined by injecting commonly encountered compounds into the LC-MS/MS system to investigate their effects on the analytes of interest, and no interference with the analytes of interest was detected. The blank containing only the mobile phase was used as a sample and subjected to LC-MS/MS analysis after the injection of a high control concentration directly in order to examine any carryover effects.

2.6. Statistical Analysis

All statistical measurements included in this work were conducted using Statistical Packages for Software Sciences version 29 purchased from IBM Corporation (Armonk, New York, NY, USA).

3. Results

3.1. Demographic Profile

Data from the 15 FCC specimens examined in this study were evaluated. In these cases, the median age of the patients was 26 years (range: 18–50 years-old, 93% were male, and 47% were aged between 21 and 30-year-old. Patients were classified into three groups according to their BMI (normal (BMI = 18–24.9, overweight (BMI = 25–30), and obese (BMI $\geq$ 30)), and almost 40% of the deceased were classified as having normal BMI. The median PMIs of the current study was 48 h, and signs of putrefaction were observed in ten out of fifteen cases in the current study (three and seven of these cases were classified as partially and heavily decomposed cases). In this study, 60% and 87% of patients had a history of drug-related disorders and polydrug pharmacies, respectively (Table 1).

Table 1. Demographic profiles of 15 patients included in this study.

Case No.	Case Information	Age	PMI	Sign of Putrefaction	Co-Ingested Substances	Location	Manner of Death	Cause of Death
1.	Deceased with history of chronic drug used was found dead in a car.	36	24	Heavily decomposed	Amphetamine	Outdoor	Accidental injury	Non-Drug related Death
2.	Fall from height, died at hospital	33	24	Non-putrefied	None	Outdoor	Accidental injury	Non-Drug related Death
3.	Poly drug intoxication, history of drug abuse	23	48	Non-putrefied	Heroin metabolites (6-monoacetylmorphine, morphine and codeine), Cocaine metabolites (Benzoylecgonine, ecgonine methyl ester), Alprazolam, Pregabalin	Indoor	Accidental overdose	Drug overdose
4.	Poly drug intoxication, history of drug abuse	23	48	Non-putrefied	Heroin metabolites (6-monoacetylmorphine, morphine and codeine), Ethanol, Alprazolam, Tramadol	Indoor	Accidental overdose	Drug overdose
5.	Gun shooting	18	24	Partially putrefied	None	Indoor	Homicidal	Non-Drug related Death
6.	Fall from height	26	72	Heavily decomposed	Methamphetamine, Amphetamine, Alprazolam, Tramadol	Outdoor	Homicidal	Non-Drug related Death
7.	Found dead on the street	40	96	Heavily decomposed	Amphetamine	Outdoor	Suicidal	Non-Drug related Death
8.	Found dead in his car	22	24	Heavily decomposed	Heroin metabolites (6-monoacetylmorphine, morphine and codeine)	Outdoor	Accidental overdose	Drug overdose

Table 1. Cont.

Case No.	Case Information	Age	PMI	Sign of Putrefaction	Co-Ingested Substances	Location	Manner of Death	Cause of Death
9.	Drug overdose	21	130	Partially putrefied	Acetone Ethanol Barbiturates Clonazepam	Indoor	Accidental overdose	Drug overdose
10.	The deceased was found hanging	22	24	Non-putrefied	Amphetamine Gabapentin Alprazolam	Indoor	Suicidal	Non-Drug related Death
11.	Drug overdose	50	320	Heavily decomposed	Amphetamine Ethanol Tramadol Lidocaine	Indoor	Accidental overdose	Drug overdose
12.	Car accident	42	72	Partially putrefied	Amphetamine	Outdoor	Accidental injury	Drug related death
13.	Found dead in his car, heavily decomposed	47	24	Heavily decomposed	Ethanol Amphetamine	Indoor	Accidental overdose	Drug related death
14.	Polydrug intoxication, history of drug abuse	21	48	Non-putrefied	Heroin metabolites (6-monoacetylmorphine, morphine and codeine) Ethanol Alprazolam Tramadol	Indoor	Accidental overdose	Drug overdose
15.	Fall from height.	37	120	Heavily decomposed	Amphetamine, Tadalafil	Indoor	Accidental injury	Drug related death

3.2. Case Samples

3.2.1. THC-COOH in FCC

FCC samples were collected from 15 postmortem cases; only THC-COOH was positive (median THC-COOH = 480 ng/mL, range concentration = 80–3010 ng/mL). THC-COOH in FCC concentrations were higher than THC-COOH concentrations in all tested specimens, with the exception of bile (Table 2 and Figure 1), and the median ratios FCC/BNaF, FCC/urine, FCC/gastric content, FCC/bile, FCC/liver, FCC/kidney, FCC/brain, FCC/stomach wall, FCC/lung, and FCC/intestine tissues were 48, 2, 0.2, 6, 4, 6, 102, 11, 5, and 10-fold, respectively.

Table 2. Summary of Δ^9-tetrahydrocannabinol in multiple postmortem specimens from 15 cases included in this study.

		Number of Cases	Median	Minimum	Maximum
Blood with Sodium Fluoride	Δ^9-tetrahydrocannabinol (THC)	10	10	102	20.0
	11-norΔ^9-THC-9-carboxylic acid	11	20.0	2.0	100.0
	11-hydroxy-Δ^9-THC	9	3.0	1.0	10.0
Fluid from Chest Cavity	THC	0	n.a. [&]	n.a.	n.a.
	11-nor-Δ^9-THC-9-carboxylic acid	15	480.0	80.0	3010.0
	11-hydroxy-Δ^9-THC	0	n.a.	n.a.	n.a.
Urine	THC	4	3.0	2.0	10.0
	11-nor-Δ^9-THC-9-carboxylic acid	10	370.0	20.0	1560.0
	11-hydroxy-Δ^9-THC	6	2.0	Tr [#]	4.0
Bile	THC	8	120.0	6.0	250.0
	11-nor-Δ^9-THC-9-carboxylic acid	13	210.0	40.0	33,000.0
	11-hydroxy-Δ^9-THC	13	110.0	3.0	1350.0
Gastric Contents	THC	10	80.0	5.0	280.0
	11-nor-Δ^9-THC-9-carboxylic acid	9	50.0	1.0	1020.0
	11-hydroxy-Δ^9-THC	4	4.0	1.0	30.0
Liver	THC	4	2.0	1.0	30.0
	11-nor-Δ^9-THC-9-carboxylic acid	14	120.0	14.0	440.0
	11-hydroxy-Δ^9-THC	2	1.0	Tr	1.0
Kidney	THC	7	2.0	1.0	70.0
	11-nor-Δ^9-THC-9-carboxylic acid	14	70.0	1.0	500.0
	11-hydroxy-Δ^9-THC	3	1.0	1.0	140.0
Brain	THC	3	20.0	14.0	20.0
	11-nor-Δ^9-THC-9-carboxylic acid	3	4.0	4.0	10.0
	11-hydroxy-Δ^9-THC	4	2.0	1.0	10.5
Stomach Wall Tissue	THC	6	30.0	4.0	470.0
	11-nor-Δ^9-THC-9-carboxylic acid	5	30.0	6.0	110.0
	11-hydroxy-Δ^9-THC	0	n.a.	n.a.	n.a.
Lung	THC	5	20.0	3.0	40.0
	11-nor-Δ^9-THC-9-carboxylic acid	5	40.0	4.0	75.0
	11-hydroxy-Δ^9-THC	1	n.a.	n.a.	n.a.
Small Intestine tissue	THC	0	n.a.	n.a.	n.a.
	11-nor-Δ^9-THC-9-carboxylic acid	4	145.0	30.0	1050.0
	11-hydroxy-Δ^9-THC	2	38.5	20.0	60.0

[&] n.a: no samples, not detected or low sample size; [#] Tr: trace concentration.

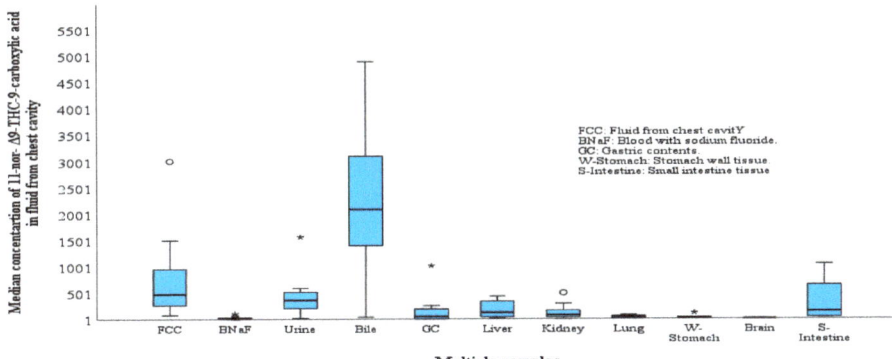

Figure 1. Concentrations of 11-nor-Δ^9-carboxy tetrahydrocannabinol in different specimens, fluid obtained from the chest and/or abdominal cavities (FCC, ng/mL), blood with sodium fluoride (ng/mL), urine (ng/mL), bile (ng/mL), gastric content (ng/mL), liver tissues (ng/g), kidney tissues (ng/g), lung tissues (ng/g), stomach wall tissues (W-Stomach) (ng/g), brain tissue (ng/g) and small intestine tissue (S-Intestine) (ng/g) of tested 15 postmortem cases. The horizontal boxes represent the median concentration ratio, and the box lengths represent the 25–75th percentile. The whiskers represent the smallest and largest value within 1.5 times the interquartile range, and circles (outlier) represent values exceeding 1.5–3 times the interquartile range.

3.2.2. Cause and Manner of Death

Table 3 shows that the differences between FCC and BNaF in accordance with the cause of death can be classified into three types: deaths solely due to drug overdose, death-related fatalities by the combination of drug use and other circumstances such as car accidents, falls from height, etc., and death unrelated to drugs such as violence and homicides. The THC-COOH concentration in the FCC was higher in drug-related deaths than in the drug-only and non-drug-related fatalities groups (Figure 2). No differences were observed between the THC-COOH concentration in both accidental overdose and accidental injury manner of deaths; the highest THC-COOH was determined in homicidal cases with 1160 ng/mL, and the lowest THC-COOH concentration was found in suicidal manner of deaths (190 ng/mL) (Figure 3). Figure 4 shows a higher median of THC-COOH in the FCC in heavy and partially putrefied cases than in non-petrified cases.

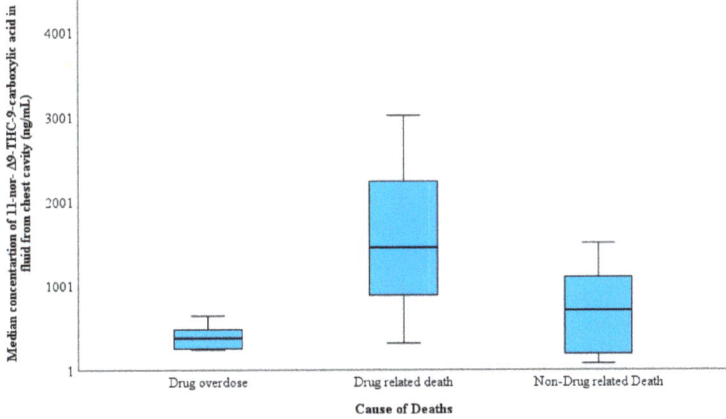

Figure 2. Variation in 11-nor-Δ^9-THC-9-carboxylic acid (THC-COOH) concentration in the fluid collected from the chest cavity in 15 cases according to the cause of death.

Table 3. Comparison between 11-nor-Δ^9-THC-9-carboxylic acid concentrations (ng/mL) in fluid from the chest cavity and blood with sodium fluoride according to cause of death, manner of death, location where the body was discovered, putrefaction, and history of drug abuse.

		Blood with Sodium Fluoride									Fluid from Chest Cavity		
		Δ^9-Tetrahydrocannabinol			11-Nor-Δ^9-THC-9-Carboxylic Acid			11-hydroxy-Δ^9-THC			11-nor-Δ^9-THC-9-Carboxylic Acid		
		NS*	Median	Range	NS*	Median	Range	NS*	Median	Range	NS*	Median	Range
Cause of Death	Drug overdose	2	15	10.0–19	3	24	17.0–103.0	2	5	3.0–10	6	378	240.0–1100.0
	Drug related death	3	7	2.0–10	3	18	2.0–40.0	2	1	0.5–1	3	1450	314.0–3010.0
	Non-Drug related Death	5	6	1.0–20	5	22	6.0–26.0	5	3	0.5–8	6	703	76.0–1500.0
Manner of Death	Accidental Overdose	3	10	7.0–20	4	32	17.0–103.0	3	3	1–7	7	476	240.0–3010.0
	Accidental injury	3	10	2.0–20	3	18	2.0–22.0	2	4	1–10	4	452	76.0–1450.0
	Homicidal	2	9	4.0–13	2	16	6.0–26.0	2	3	n.a	2	1158	816.2–1500.0
	Suicidal	2	3	1.2–6	2	22	n.a	2	1	n.a	2	645	n.a.
Location of death	Indoor	6	9	1.2–20	7	21	6.0–103.0	5	3	1–7	8	461	189.0–3010.0
	Outdoor	4	9	1.7–20	4	23	2.0–26.0	4	3	1–10	7	480	76.0–1500.0
Putrefaction	Non-putrefied	4	15	1.2–20	4	22	17.0–103.0	4	5	0.5–8	5	240	76.0–480.0
	Partially putrefied	2	3	1.7–4	3	6	2.0–24.0	2	2	n.a	3	642	314.0–816.2
	Heavy putrefied	4	9	6–13	4	25	18.0–40.0	3	2	0.5–3	7	1100	255.0–3010.0
Poly drug used	No	2	12	4.0–20	2	14	6.0–22.0	2	6	3.0–8	2	446	76.0–816.2
	Yes	8	9	1.2–20	9	23	2.0–103.0	7	2	0.5–7	13	480	189.0–3010.0
History of drug of abuse	No	4	9	1.2–20	4	22	6.0–26.0	4	3	1–8	6	535	76.0–1500.0
	Yes	6	9	1.7–19	7	23	2.0–103.0	5	2	1–7	9	476	240.0–3010.0

* NS: Number of samples, n.a: Not available.

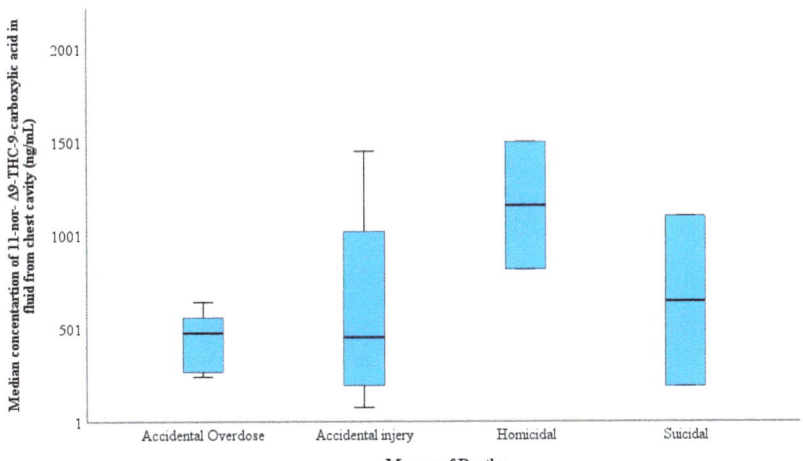

Figure 3. Variation in 11-nor-Δ^9-THC-9-carboxylic acid concentration in the fluid collected from the chest cavity in the 15 cases according to the manner of death.

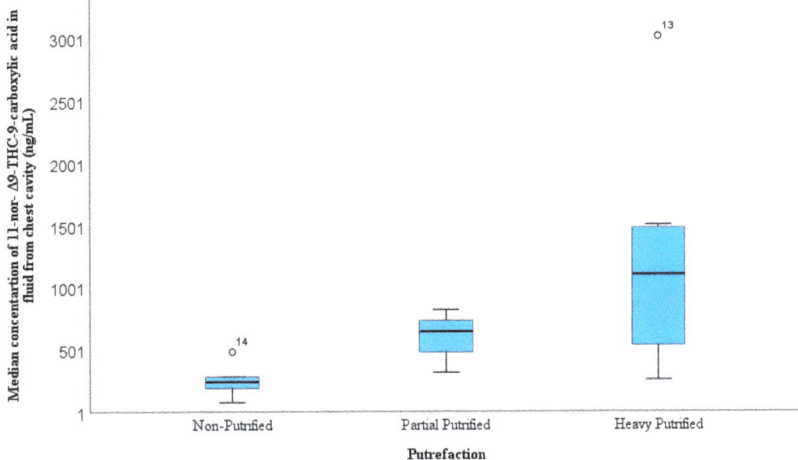

Figure 4. Variation in 11-nor-Δ^9-THC-9-carboxylic acid concentration in the fluid collected from the chest cavity in 15 cases according to the degree of putrefaction.

3.2.3. History of Drug Abuse, PMIs, and BMI

The relationship between the THC-COOH concentration in the FCC and history of drug abuse showed no significant differences (Table 3). The most obvious differences were observed in the PMIs group, in which higher concentrations were observed with longer PMI times. This could be explained by postmortem redistribution from the surrounding organs. Moreover, decreasing the water content in the case of putrefaction led to the concentration of analytes in the FCC. This is supported by the high level of THC-COOH in heavily decomposed (1100 ng/mL) cases, followed by partially putrefied cases (642 ng/mL), in comparison to non-purified cases (240 ng/mL). Differences in THC-COOH in the FCC were not observed between the BMI groups in comparison with THC-COOH in the BNaF normal BMI group level than in the overweight and obese groups.

4. Discussion

Few studies have discussed the post-mortem data on THC, THC-OH, and THC-COOH in autopsy samples. Kemp et al. [16] reported 55 cases related to cannabis use in a series of cases of deaths related to fatal aviation accidents in the USA. This study revealed the usefulness of using alternative specimens, particularly lung tissue, in postmortem cannabinoid analysis. Saenz et al. found that the use of alternative specimens is useful when severe trauma is associated with accidents in case no blood is available. In that study, vitreous humor, brain, spleen, muscle, liver, lung, kidney, bile, heart, urine, and blood were found to be suitable alternatives or supplemental choices for qualitative cannabinoid detection [11]. Comparable conclusions were reported by Cliburn et al., in which ten pilots were involved in airplane crashes [2]. Postmortem details of cannabinoid testing in multiple body fluids and tissue analyses in forensic toxicology cases unrelated to aviation accidents have rarely been reported. Al-Asmari reported 32 cases that tested positive for cannabinoids. In that study, multiple postmortem specimens, including body and tissue samples of interest, were investigated [15]. These studies identified alternative specimens suitable for routine postmortem analysis of THC and its metabolites. These studies were limited by their small sample sizes, and no correlation was found between cannabinoids and their metabolites when multiple postmortem specimens were compared.

While blood is frequently employed as a specimen in forensic toxicology investigations, it may sometimes be unavailable owing to circumstances such as fatal accidents or putrefaction [2,8,16]. In this study, non-blood samples, especially FCC, were analyzed, and because this is the first report of this type of specimen, other bodily and tissue specimen results for the same subjects were compared with the FCC results. FCC was found to be positive at higher concentrations than most matrices analyzed in postmortem cases, except for bile, which agrees with previously reported bile concentrations in ten fatally injured pilots [2,14]. The FCC samples were liquid, easy to manipulate, and were extracted using the same procedure as the blood samples. The blood procedure was chosen because of the similar nature of the samples and the use of blood calibration curves for quantification of THC-COOH in the FCC. According to ANSI/ASB guidelines [19], it is acceptable to use a whole-blood calibration curve to quantify other postmortem bodily fluids and tissues. Although these matrices are different in terms of their viscosity, protein content, and ability to pass through SPE cartridges, a full validation of each analyte of interest in each matrix of interest may be time consuming and labor intensive, and because of the availability of samples in such unusual specimens for testing such as FCC. Another option is to adapt different calibration curves for different samples for quantification and used a control from the FACA with each batch, taking into consideration in these matrices, which is logically much higher in FCC than in blood; this is also the case with drugs and different metabolites. Therefore, a higher ULOQ of 1000 ng/mL BNaF was applied.

The importance of the FCC matrix comes from the nature of the cases, as most are traumatic, violent, or putrefied cases in which non-blood or biological fluid is available or suitable for analysis. For example, in putrefied cases, solid tissues such as the liver, lung, kidney, and brain can be tested, and their extraction is usually labor- and time-consuming compared to testing bodily fluid specimens. THC and THC-OH were rarely observed in solid tissues, and only THC-COOH was easily detected, which is similar to the result from the FCC. In Kemp et al. [16] and in other study [14], THC together with THC-COOH were determined in many specimens, including solid tissues. In that study, liver and kidney specimens showed a positive result for these analytes. In a comparable manner to this work, THC-COOH was determined in the liver and kidney, which agrees with earlier reports [11,14–16]. In these case study reports, THC-COOH levels ranged from 8.0 to 3894 ng/g in liver tissues and from 3 to 1774 ng/mL in kidney tissues. In contrast, the THC was negative in most cases, which agrees with the current study. The detection of THC-COOH only in most liver and kidney tissues can be explained by its role in cannabinoid metabolism and excretion from the body, as THC and its metabolites are conjugated to be eliminated in urine. THC-COOH-glucuronide degrades to THC-COOH in vivo without the need for a hydrolysis procedure during extraction, which enhances its content in these solid tissues and transfers it to surrounding bodily fluids and tissues with long PMI if tissues are not subjected to proper storage prior to death [9,15,20,21]. In a similar study on morphine conjugate metabolites, glucuronide metabolites were deconjugated to form their free forms if not immediately subjected to proper storage conditions, even without hydrolysis. This was much more obvious for analytes of interest in internal tissues, for example, in liver and kidney tissues [22]. Fluids from the chest cavity can be contaminated by postmortem interval time (PMI) and postmortem redistribution of some drugs. Postmortem changes after death could also increase the concentration of drugs, or some drugs could be degraded or evaporated [23].

In addition, the detection of free metabolites using alkaline or enzymatic procedures or instead a direct determination of conjugated metabolites of THC and its metabolite procedures has been reported, and there is always a difference between free drugs obtained using different hydrolysis methods or direct analysis [9,20]. Gronewold and Skopp [14] developed a method for the direct measurement of THC glucuronide metabolites without any hydrolysis procedure. In that study, in addition to THC metabolites, only THC-COOH-glucuronide was tested, as other glucuronide metabolites (THC-OH-glucuronide and THC-glucuronide) were not available commercially. In the report by Gronewold and Skopp, an obviously higher concentration of THC-COOH-glucuronide was found in all five cases included in their study, whereas in some cases, THC and its metabolites THC-OH were either not detected or detected at trace levels. This suggests that THC and THC-OH are significantly conjugated, which requires hydrolysis to obtain their free form, mirroring the process observed for THC-COOH. Consequently, an effective hydrolysis method is required to separate THC from THC-OH. In contrast, the free forms of these analytes were reported after alkaline hydrolysis in liver and kidney tissues, although they were present at trace levels [15,16]. Saenz et al. conducted enzymatic hydrolysis for their analysis and discovered that these analytes could be detected in liver and kidney samples [11].

As no THC or THC-OH was detected in FCC, the source of THC-COOH detected in FCC could be derived from the surrounding organs due to postmortem redistribution or contamination due to postmortem changes after death. This could also be explained by the slow transport of THC and its metabolites from the blood to organs and the lag in distribution between the blood, surrounding organs, and FCC. However, THC-COOH, which is stored in adipose tissue, could be a major source of THC-COOH found in the FCC. Other alternative specimens, such as bile, gastric contents, brain tissue, stomach wall tissues, and lung tissues, were found to be perfect matrices for the measurement of THC and THC-OH in the current study and previous investigations [2,11,15]. Al-Asmari suggested that the detection of THC in the stomach wall specimens and in the lung specimens can be justified by the influence of the route of administration as cannabinoids are smoked, thereby increasing direct contact to these tissues, thereby increasing the likelihood of THC detection in these tissues [15]. Moreover, this may be because they undergo cycles of enterohepatic movement from the liver, the site of THC, and THC-OH metabolism, in which these analytes are reabsorbed by gastric contents, which increases their concentration.

As we discuss cannabinoid use, even when using blood THC concentrations, it is still not possible to distinguish between recent and chronic use. It is believed that the concentration of cannabinoids varies depending on how often cannabinoids are consumed; however, some studies found that THC and THC-COOH could still be detected in blood up to seven days after cessation of marijuana administration [11,24]. This is because of the nature of analyte metabolism, which is deposited in adipose tissues and released into the bloodstream for a longer period when individuals do not smoke [11]. Nevertheless, in a recent study, the distribution of THC and its metabolites differed depending on renal function, body mass index, body composition, and gender [17]. Therefore, if the detection of THC can be used to confirm its recent use, this is misleading, and it is not recommended in toxicology investigations. The correlation between blood and other specimens is always poor owing to several issues such as the water content and the weight of the tissues constantly changing during the putrefying process, PMI, and postmortem redistribution phenomena, which can also affect FCC testing. However, alternative specimens can be used to provide complementary information to blood, and in cases where no blood or other traditional samples such as urine, vitreous humor, liver, and other traditionally used specimens are available at postmortem investigation [11]. Cliburn et al. believed that information obtained from these complementary specimens may add useful information to the scarce real postmortem cannabinoid case study available in the literature and advise suitable biological and tissue matrices for investigating cannabinoid-related deaths [2].

One of the limitations of using FCC is the small sample size and analysis of this specimen directly without using a hydrolysis procedure. However, in agreement with most previous investigations, poor correlations were often obtained between THC metabolite concentrations in the blood, body, and tissue specimens. This can be attributed to the lack of information regarding the route, time, and dosage of cannabinoids administered [2].

5. Conclusions

This is the first postmortem study to report THC-COOH in the FCC in real samples. FCC is a promising sample, as in some cases where blood and other biological fluids are unavailable, it can provide information regarding cannabinoid administration, considering that contamination from the surrounding tissues cannot be excluded. The impact of using FCC as an alternative sample is to provide suitable and homogenate specimens appropriate for testing analytes of interest that can be extracted easily compared to solid tissue specimens that are always tested in cases where no blood is available. Nevertheless, the value of the FCC matrix comes from the nature of the cases tested in this project, as most are traumatic, violent, or putrefied cases in which non-blood or biological fluid is available or suitable for analysis. The limitations of using FCC were the small sample size and direct analysis of this specimen without using a hydrolysis procedure, and more research is needed with different hydrolysis methods to investigate the presence of other cannabinoid metabolites.

Author Contributions: Conceptualization, T.A.Z., A.I.A.-A. and H.A.; methodology, A.I.A.-A., H.A. and A.E.A.; software, A.I.A.-A.; validation, A.I.A.-A. and A.A.-S.; formal analysis, A.A.-S., H.A. and A.E.A.; investigation, T.A.Z., A.I.A.-A. and H.A.; resources, H.A., A.E.A. and A.A.-S.; data curation, A.I.A.-A., H.A. and A.E.A.; writing—original draft preparation, A.I.A.-A. and T.A.Z.; writing—review and editing, T.A.Z. and A.I.A.-A.; visualization, A.I.A.-A.; supervision, A.I.A.-A., H.A. and T.A.Z.; project administration, T.A.Z. and H.A. All authors have read and agreed to the published version of the manuscript.

Funding: The research was funded by Institutional Fund Projects under grant no. IFPIP: 459-142-1443.

Institutional Review Board Statement: The study was conducted in accordance with the Declaration of Helsinki and approved by the Ethics Committee of the Ministry of Health (MOH), Jeddah Health Affairs, in the Kingdom of Saudi Arabia, research code: ethical approval no. H-02-J-002.

Informed Consent Statement: Not applicable.

Data Availability Statement: The data underlying this article will be shared upon reasonable request by the corresponding authors.

Acknowledgments: The authors gratefully acknowledge technical and financial support provided by the Ministry of Education and King Abdulaziz University, DSR, Jeddah, Saudi Arabia. The authors would like to thank all the staff at the Forensic Toxicology Department-Jeddah Poison Control and Forensic Medical Chemistry Center for supporting this work.

Conflicts of Interest: The authors declare no conflict of interest.

References

1. Chandra, S.; Radwan, M.M.; Majumdar, C.G.; Church, J.C.; Freeman, T.P.; ElSohly, M.A. New Trends in Cannabis Potency in USA and Europe during the Last Decade (2008–2017). *Eur. Arch. Psychiatry Clin. Neurosci.* **2019**, *269*, 5–15. [CrossRef] [PubMed]
2. Cliburn, K.D.; Huestis, M.A.; Wagner, J.R.; Kemp, P.M. Cannabinoid Distribution in Fatally-Injured Pilots' Postmortem Fluids and Tissues. *Forensic Sci. Int.* **2021**, *329*, 111075. [CrossRef]
3. Lewis, B.; Fleeger, T.; Judge, B.; Riley, B.; Jones, J.S. Acute Toxicity Associated with Cannabis Edibles Following Decriminalization of Marijuana in Michigan. *Am. J. Emerg. Med.* **2021**, *46*, 732–735. [CrossRef] [PubMed]
4. Wickens, C.M.; Ialomiteanu, A.R.; di Ciano, P.; Stoduto, G.; Mann, R.E. Use of Cannabis and/or Prescription Opioids among Adult Drivers in Ontario, Canada: Prevalence and Association with Motor Vehicle Collisions. *J. Transp. Health* **2021**, *22*, 101091. [CrossRef]
5. Shirah, B.H.; Ahmed, M.M. The Use of Cannabis for Medical Purposes in the Arab World. *Med. Cannabis Cannabinoids* **2021**, *4*, 72–74. [CrossRef] [PubMed]
6. Al-Asmari, A.I.; Alharbi, H.; Al-Zahrani, A.E.; Zughaibi, T.A. Heroin-Related Fatalities in Jeddah, Saudi Arabia, between 2008 and 2018. *Toxics* **2023**, *11*, 248. [CrossRef]
7. Al-Asmari, A.I. Methamphetamine-Related Postmortem Cases in Jeddah, Saudi Arabia. *Forensic Sci. Int.* **2021**, *321*, 110746. [CrossRef]
8. Cliburn, K.D.; Huestis, M.A.; Wagner, J.R.; Kemp, P.M. Identification and Quantification of Cannabinoids in Postmortem Fluids and Tissues by Liquid Chromatography-Tandem Mass Spectrometry. *J. Chromatogr. A* **2021**, *1652*, 462345. [CrossRef] [PubMed]
9. Al-Asmari, A.I. Method for Postmortem Quantification of Δ^9-Tetrahydrocannabinol and Metabolites Using LC-MS-MS. *J. Anal. Toxicol.* **2019**, *43*, 703–719. [CrossRef]
10. Ashton, C.H. Pharmacology and Effects of Cannabis: A Brief Review. *Br. J. Psychiatry* **2001**, *178*, 101–106. [CrossRef] [PubMed]
11. Saenz, S.R.; Lewis, R.J.; Angier, M.K.; Wagner, J.R. Postmortem Fluid and Tissue Concentrations of THC, 11-OH-THC and THC-COOH. *J. Anal. Toxicol.* **2017**, *41*, 508–516. [CrossRef] [PubMed]
12. Fabritius, M.; Staub, C.; Mangin, P.; Giroud, C. Distribution of Free and Conjugated Cannabinoids in Human Bile Samples. *Forensic Sci. Int.* **2012**, *223*, 114–118. [CrossRef] [PubMed]
13. Lemos, N.P.; Ingle, E.A. Cannabinoids in Postmortem Toxicology. *J. Anal. Toxicol.* **2011**, *35*, 394–401. [CrossRef] [PubMed]
14. Gronewold, A.; Skopp, G. A Preliminary Investigation on the Distribution of Cannabinoids in Man. *Forensic Sci. Int.* **2011**, *210*, e7–e11. [CrossRef] [PubMed]
15. Al-Asmari, A.I. Method for Postmortem Tissue Quantification of Δ^9-Tetrahydrocannabinol and Metabolites Using LC–MS-MS. *J. Anal. Toxicol.* **2020**, *44*, 718–733. [CrossRef]
16. Kemp, P.M.; Cardona, P.S.; Chaturvedi, A.K.; Soper, J.W. Distribution of Δ^9-Tetrahydrocannabinol and 11-Nor-9-Carboxy-Δ^9-Tetrahydrocannabinol Acid in Postmortem Biological Fluids and Tissues From Pilots Fatally Injured in Aviation Accidents. *J. Forensic Sci.* **2015**, *60*, 942–949. [CrossRef]
17. Zughaibi, T.A.; Al-Qumsani, L.; Mirza, A.A.; Almostady, A.; Basrawi, J.; Tabrez, S.; Alsolami, F.; Al-Makki, R.; Al-Ghamdi, S.; Al-Ghamdi, A.; et al. Comparison between Blood, Non-Blood Fluids and Tissue Specimens for the Analysis of Cannabinoid Metabolites in Cannabis-Related Post-Mortem Cases. *Forensic Sci.* **2023**, *3*, 330–344. [CrossRef]
18. Matuszewski, B.K.; Constanzer, M.L.; Chavez-Eng, C.M. Strategies for the Assessment of Matrix Effect in Quantitative Bioanalytical Methods Based on HPLC-MS/MS. *Anal. Chem.* **2003**, *75*, 3019–3030. [CrossRef]
19. *ANSI/ASB Standard 036*; Method Validation in Forensic Toxicology. American Academy of Forensic Sciences Standards Board: Colorado Springs, CO, USA, 2019.
20. Kemp, P.M.; Abukhalaf, I.K.; Manno, J.E.; Manno, B.R.; Alford, D.D.; Mc Williams, M.E.; Nixon, F.E.; Fitzgerald, M.J.; Reeves, R.R.; Wood, M.J. Cannabinoids in Humans. Ii. the Influence of Three Methods of Hydrolysis on the Conentration of Thc and Two Metabolites in Urine. *J. Anal. Toxicol.* **1995**, *19*, 292–298. [CrossRef]
21. Duflou, J.; Darke, S.; Easson, J. Morphine Concentrations in Stomach Contents of Intravenous Opioid Overdose Deaths. *J. Forensic Sci.* **2009**, *54*, 1181–1184. [CrossRef]
22. Moriya, F.; Hashimoto, Y. Distribution of Free and Conjugated Morphine in Body Fluids and Tissues in a Fatal Heroin Overdose: Is Conjugated Morphine Stable in Postmortem Specimens? *J. Forensic Sci.* **1997**, *42*, 736–740. [CrossRef] [PubMed]
23. Skopp, G. Preanalytic Aspects in Postmortem Toxicology. *Forensic Sci. Int.* **2004**, *142*, 75–100. [CrossRef]
24. Karschner, E.L.; Schwilke, E.W.; Lowe, R.H.; Darwin, W.D.; Pope, H.G.; Herning, R.; Cadet, J.L.; Huestis, M.A. Do Δ^9-Tetrahydrocannabinol Concentrations Indicate Recent Use in Chronic Cannabis Users? *Addiction* **2009**, *104*, 2041–2048. [CrossRef] [PubMed]

Disclaimer/Publisher's Note: The statements, opinions and data contained in all publications are solely those of the individual author(s) and contributor(s) and not of MDPI and/or the editor(s). MDPI and/or the editor(s) disclaim responsibility for any injury to people or property resulting from any ideas, methods, instructions or products referred to in the content.

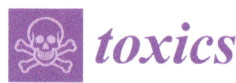

Article

Heroin-Related Fatalities in Jeddah, Saudi Arabia, between 2008 and 2018

Ahmed I. Al-Asmari [1,2,*], Hassan Alharbi [3], Abdulnasser E. Al-Zahrani [3] and Torki A. Zughaibi [2,4,*]

1. Laboratory Department, Ministry of Health, King Abdul-Aziz Hospital, Jeddah 21442, Saudi Arabia
2. King Fahd Medical Research Center, King Abdulaziz University, Jeddah 21589, Saudi Arabia
3. Poison Control and Forensic Chemistry Center, Ministry of Health, Jeddah 21176, Saudi Arabia
4. Department of Medical Laboratory Sciences, Faculty of Applied Medical Sciences, King Abdulaziz University, Jeddah 21589, Saudi Arabia
* Correspondence: aial-asmari2@moh.gov.sa or ahmadalasmari@yahoo.com (A.I.A.-A.); taalzughaibi@kau.edu.sa (T.A.Z.)

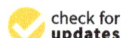

Citation: Al-Asmari, A.I.; Alharbi, H.; Al-Zahrani, A.E.; Zughaibi, T.A. Heroin-Related Fatalities in Jeddah, Saudi Arabia, between 2008 and 2018. *Toxics* 2023, 11, 248. https://doi.org/10.3390/toxics11030248

Academic Editor: Eric J. F. Franssen

Received: 21 January 2023
Revised: 20 February 2023
Accepted: 27 February 2023
Published: 6 March 2023

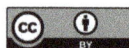

Copyright: © 2023 by the authors. Licensee MDPI, Basel, Switzerland. This article is an open access article distributed under the terms and conditions of the Creative Commons Attribution (CC BY) license (https://creativecommons.org/licenses/by/4.0/).

Abstract: To date, epidemiological studies have not evaluated heroin-related deaths in the Middle East and North African regions, especially Saudi Arabia. All heroin-related postmortem cases reported at the Jeddah Poison Control Center (JPCC) over a 10-year period (21 January 2008 to 31 July 2018) were reviewed. In addition, liquid chromatography electrospray ionization tandem mass spectrometry (LC/ESI-MS/MS) was utilized to determine the 6-monoacetylmorphine (6-MAM), 6-acetylcodeine (6-AC), morphine (MOR), and codeine contents in unhydrolyzed postmortem specimens. Ninety-seven heroin-related deaths were assessed in this study, and they represented 2% of the total postmortem cases at the JPCC (median age, 38; 98% male). In the blood, urine, vitreous humor, and bile samples, the median morphine concentrations were 280 ng/mL, 1400 ng/mL, 90 ng/mL, and 2200 ng/mL, respectively; 6-MAM was detected in 60%, 100%, 99%, and 59% of the samples, respectively; and 6-AC was detected in 24%, 68%, 50%, and 30% of the samples, respectively. The highest number of deaths (33% of total cases) was observed in the 21–30 age group. In addition, 61% of cases were classified as "rapid deaths," while 24% were classified as "delayed deaths." The majority (76%) of deaths were accidental; 7% were from suicide; 5% were from homicide; and 11% were undetermined. This is the first epidemiological study to investigate heroin-related fatalities in Saudi Arabia and the Middle East and North African region. The rate of heroin-related deaths in Jeddah remained stable but increased slightly at the end of the study period. Most patients were heroin-dependent abusers and from the middle-aged group. The availability of urine, vitreous humor, and bile specimens provided valuable information regarding the opioids that were administered and the survival time following heroin injection.

Keywords: forensic toxicology; opiates; opioids; LC-MS/MS; postmortem

1. Introduction

The abuse of heroin (diamorphine, acetomorphine, and diacetylmorphine) remains a major cause of death worldwide. For example, an estimated 62 million people used opioids for non-medical purposes in 2019 (1.2% of the global population), with half using heroin or opium [1]. The primary cause of heroin-related deaths is overdose [2–4], while indirect causes of death include infectious diseases, such as human immunodeficiency virus (HIV) and hepatitis, and sepsis associated with intravenous injection [2]. The latest United Nations Office on Drug and Crime (UNDOC) report indicated that in 2019, heroin trafficking occurred in ninety-nine countries [1]. According to a recent report from the European Union, heroin is the most abused opioid. In 2019, 85% of the drug-related deaths in Europe were caused by one or more opioids [5]. Currently, North America is experiencing a sharp rise in heroin users, with an increase of approximately 150% from 2007 to 2017 [1]. In the United States, Evans et al. analyzed drug residues from needle-exchange syringes and found that heroin was the second most detected controlled substance [6]. In the last UNODC report published in 2022 [1], it was stated that although heroin is not the primary cause of death related to opioids in the USA, it is still causing fatalities via ingestion, either intentionally or accidentally. It has been estimated that 9.5 million people were using opioids non-medically in the past year in the USA. Almost 98% of them were using pharmaceutical opioids non-medically; in this period, 9.5% were using heroin, and 7.4% used both heroin and pharmaceutical opioids. Based on another report [7], heroin alone as a cause of death seems to be declining; however, heroin-related fatalities have been increasing in terms of deaths in that region. Heroin found in such cases was allegedly ingested accidentally, as most cases were also fentanyl-related fatalities, and this is most likely due to the mixing of heroin with fentanyl in the black market. According to a UNODC report, heroin is still the predominant opioid used in many Asian countries, such as India and Pakistan. In 2018, 23 million Indians were estimated to use opioids, and heroin was the most frequently used drug among the population. In contrast, a 50% decline in heroin use has been reported among registered drug users in China [1].

In the Middle East and North African (MENA) region, principally in the Arabian Gulf region, heroin is reported in the media as a symbol of drug addiction. However, heroin-related fatalities have rarely been reported in scientific literature from this region. Thus, little is known about heroin-related deaths, and most studies in the Arabian Gulf region are outdated [8,9]. Al-Matrouk et al. reviewed these studies and found that they were mostly survey-based and lacked laboratory-based research; thus, these studies did not actually describe the real situation of drug abuse patterns in these countries [10].

In Saudi Arabia, alcohol and drug use are prohibited by law and denounced based on social and religious perspectives [11,12]. Thus, Saudi drug use is poorly understood. In one study, the abuse of heroin in recent years appeared to decrease or was not reported in certain regions of Saudi Arabia, such as the Al-Qassim region [13]. In contrast, heroin was the second most detected drug at Jeddah's Addiction Hospital [8]. In the eastern region of Saudi Arabia, 49% of overdose deaths were related to opiates (116 out of 249 drug-related deaths) in an 8-year period from 1990 to 1997 [14]. However, in that study, postmortem details were not reported; thus, whether heroin or codeine was the main opioid was not determined.

Heroin is unstable in biological specimens and rarely identified in postmortem cases [15]. Alternatively, its biomarkers (6-monoacetylmorphine (6-MAM) and 6-acetylcodeine (6-AC)) provide sufficient evidence to demonstrate whether heroin was the opioid administered and whether death occurred shortly following ingestion. 6-MAM has a short half-life of ~40 min before converting to morphine [16]. However, 6-AC metabolism and its role in heroin-related fatalities have rarely been reported [17,18]. In cases of death, if sample collection is delayed, then heroin biomarkers will be converted to morphine and codeine. Morphine is an active metabolite of heroin with a much longer half-life than heroin and 6-MAM, whereas codeine is formed by 6-AC degradation [2]. In fact, 6-MAM, morphine, and morphine metabolites have frequently been reported in heroin-related deaths, whereas the presence of 6-AC in postmortem cases has rarely been reported [19,20], which may be due to its short half-life, instability under storage conditions, and incredibly low concentrations in deceased specimens [15,20]. To the best of our knowledge, no epidemiological studies have reported 6-MAM and 6-AC together in a postmortem specimen in heroin-related fatalities.

The patterns of heroin-related deaths are poorly understood in the MENA region. Thus, up-to-date epidemiological studies to reveal heroin-related fatalities and explore the problem of heroin abuse are a crucial task. As Jeddah is one of the major cities in Saudi Arabia (4 million population), this paper reports the first epidemiological study evaluating heroin-related deaths in Jeddah City, Saudi Arabia, between 2008 and 2018 and investigates whether metabolites of heroin found in various bodily fluid samples can be used to identify the type of opioid ingested and the time of death after administration.

Such toxicological information is crucial for providing knowledge on the trends in illegal drug use and planning initiatives to reduce accidents and deaths among drug users.

2. Materials and Methods

2.1. Reagents and Standards

Morphine, morphine-d3, 6-MAM, 6-monoacetylmorphine-d3 (6-MAM-d3), codeine, codeine-d3, and 6-AC were purchased from Lipomed (Arlesheim, Switzerland). Methanol (HPLC grade), acetonitrile (HPLC grade), ammonium carbonate, formic acid, and ammonium hydroxide were obtained from BDH (Poole, UK). Ammonium formate was obtained from Sigma-Aldrich (Steinheim, Germany). Clean Screen® solid phase extraction (SPE) cartridges (CSDAU203) were obtained from United Chemical Technologies (Bristol, PA, USA).

2.2. Solid Phase Extraction (SPE)

One milliliter of each specimen was placed in a glass test tube, which was then spiked with 50 µL of the internal standard (containing 50 µg/mL of 6-MAM-d3, morphine-d3, and codeine-d3). The mixture was then mixed and vortexed for at least 10 s. Next, 2 mL of 0.1 M phosphate buffer (pH 6) was added to the samples, mixed, and centrifuged for 10 min at 3500 rpm. Before loading the samples into the SPE cartridges, the samples were prepared for SPE by adding 2 mL of methanol, 2 mL of deionized water ($D.H_2O$), and 2 mL of 0.1 M phosphate buffer adjusted to pH 6. The sample mixture was then loaded onto the SPE column using gravity. Next, the cartridges were washed by adding 1 mL of $D.H_2O$, followed by 1 mL of acetic acid (0.1 M), and then dried under vacuum for 5 min. The third washing step was completed by adding 2 mL of hexane. Two elution steps were performed: the first elution (A) was performed by adding 2 mL hexane/ethyl acetate (1:1, v/v). Next, the elution tubes were removed, and the SPE cartridges were washed using 3 mL of methanol and then dried under full vacuum for 2 min. The second elution (B) was performed by adding 3 mL of dichloromethane/isopropanol/ammonium hydroxide (78:20:2, v/v) to each cartridge. Both fractions were collected in a glass evaporation tube and evaporated to dryness using nitrogen. Finally, 200 µL of the initial mobile phase was added to the final extracts and subjected to liquid chromatography tandem mass spectrometry (LC-MS/MS) using an injection volume of 1.0 µL.

2.3. LC-MS/MS Systems

Two different LC-MS/MS systems were used to analyze the heroin biomarkers, morphine, and codeine. The first system included a Thermo Finnigan LCQ Fleet ion trap instrument equipped with a Surveyor LC system interface (Thermo Finnigan, San Jose, USA) equipped with electrospray ionization (ESI+) and selective reaction monitoring modes. Analytes were separated using a Synergy Polar RP column (150 × 2.0 mm, 4 µm particle size, Phenomenex, Torrance, CA, USA) equipped with a guard column with identical packing material (4 × 2.0 mm, Phenomenex, Torrance, CA, USA). The column oven and auto-sampler tray temperatures were kept at 30 °C and 4 °C, respectively. The gradient mobile phase consisted of ammonium formate buffer (10 mM, pH 3) as mobile phase A and an organic modifier of 100% acetonitrile as mobile phase B, with a flow rate of 0.3 mL/min for the whole run. The gradient program was initiated by applying 3% B for 3 min, which was increased to 15% over the next 5 min, 26% over the next 7 min, 80% over the next 13 min, and 95% over the next two min. After 27 min, the initial mobile phase was applied for 3 min. Data were acquired and managed using the Xcalibur system (Version 2.07 SP1, Thermo Finnigan, San Jose, USA).

The second LC-MS/MS analysis was performed according to a previously reported method [20]. Brifly, LC-MS/MS with a triple quadrupole mass spectrometer (Shimadzu LCMS-8050, Kyoto, Japan), (+)ESI, and a Shimadzu Nexera UHPLC system were used for the analysis of 6-MAM, 6-AC, morphine, and codeine. Analytes of interest were separated using a phenyl LC-column (Raptor Biphenyl column (50 × 3.0 mm, 2.7 µm, Restek,

USA) fitted with a guard column with a similar chemistry (Raptor Biophenyl column (5.0 × 3.0 mm, 2.7 µm, Restek, USA). The gradient condition mobile phase consisted of ammonium formate (10 mM, pH 3, mobile phase A) and 100% methanol (mobile phase B), and the flow rate was 0.3 mL/min for the whole run. The mobile phase gradient elution started with 3% B during the first minute and then increased to 5% within 1 min and 95% over the next 13 min. The initial mobile phase was then applied for 1 min and maintained for the next 4 min to re-equilibrate and prepare the column for the next injection. The LC-MS/MS parameters are listed in Table S1. Data were acquired and managed using LabSolution software (version 5.75, Shimadzu, Kyoto, Japan). The LC-MS/MS parameters are listed in Table 1.

Table 1. Liquid chromatography electrospray ionization tandem mass spectrometry (LC-MS/MS) data for heroin biomarkers, morphine, and codeine.

Analytes [&]	Internal Standards	RT * (min)	Quantifier Ion	Qualifier Ion	RT (min)	Quantifier Ion	Qualifier Ion
			LC-MS 8050			LCQ Fleet	
Analytes							
6-MAM	6-MAM-d3	6.9	m/z = 328−165	m/z = 328−221	15.1	m/z1 = 328−211	m/z = 328−268
6-MAM-d3 [#]	-	7.0	m/z = 331-165	m/z = 331-221	15.1	m/z = 331-165	m/z = 331-221
6-AC	Codeine-d3	9.3	m/z = 342-225	m/z = 342-165	19.0	m/z = 342-225	m/z = 342-282
Morphine	Morphine-d3	4.7	m/z = 286-165	m/z = 286-153	8.4	m/z = 286-201	m/z = 286-229
Morphine-d3 [#]	-	4.6	m/z = 289-165	m/z = 289-153	8.2	m/z = 289-201	m/z = 289-229
Codeine	Codeine-d3	6.8	m/z = 300-165	m/z = 300-44	13.9	m/z = 300-215	m/z = 300-243
Codeine-d3 [#]	-	6.7	m/z = 303-165	m/z = 300-199	13.9	m/z = 303-215	m/z = 300-243

[&] Analytes: 6-monoacetylmorphine (6-MAM), 6-acetylcodeine (6-AC), RT *: Retention time. [#] Internal standard.

2.4. Case Samples

2.4.1. Ethical Approval

This study was approved by the IRB committee of Jeddah Health Affairs, Ministry of Health, Jeddah, Saudi Arabia (research no: #A00221; approval no: A00187).

2.4.2. Sample Collection

Blood samples were collected from the subclavian site in tubes containing 1% sodium fluoride (BNaF). Vitreous humor fluid was collected in gray tubes containing sodium fluoride, and urine and bile samples were stored in a plain container without any preservative. All samples were stored frozen (at −20 °C) until analysis. Autopsy samples were thawed to obtain them and refrozen until use. Blood samples were obtained for 84 postmortem cases (87%), urine samples were obtained for 74 cases (76%), vitreous humor samples were obtained from two eyes in 70 cases (72%), and bile specimens were obtained for 27 cases (28%).

2.4.3. Data Collecting for Post-Mortem Cases

All postmortem body fluids and tissues collected for forensic toxicology investigations are analyzed for commonly abused drugs and reported, and they are also assessed based on requests by forensic pathologists. All heroin-related postmortem cases reported at the Jeddah Poison Control and Medical Chemistry Center (JPCC) over the last 10-years (21 January 2008 to 31 July 2018) were reviewed. The 6-MAM, 6-AC, morphine, and codeine contents were reviewed, and case details were collected from the online Forensic Toxicology Jeddah Reports Database. The search was conducted between February 2015 and July 2018. Data before February 2015 was manually collected from JPCC archive files. Cases positive for heroin use were reviewed and included in this investigation according to the inclusion/exclusion criteria mentioned below. Ninety-seven cases reported during the study period were included.

2.4.4. Inclusion/Exclusion Criteria

The same criteria applied in our previous study were used in the current study [21]. The most important criteria included the detection of 6-MAM in blood samples available for testing or in any alternative samples, particularly vitreous humor, urine, and bile.

2.4.5. Other Toxicological Investigations

All postmortem cases, irrespective of the manner of death, were screened using a common immunoassay reagent. The second step was to search for other concomitant drugs using general unknown screening approaches (GUS), (known as systemic toxicological analysis, or STA) by gas chromatography (GC) coupled to a flame ionization detector (FID), gas chromatography coupled to mass spectrometry (GC-MS), and LC-MS/MS.

The analysis methods were all fully validated using international guidelines for forensic investigation [22], and a selectivity study was conducted that included additional toxicology testing for drugs and their metabolites that are commonly detected in postmortem forensic toxicology. The analyses used whole blood, urine, or tissue specimens when other body fluid samples were not available. STA includes immunoassay testing, which employs two separate instruments: alcohol testing using GC-Headspace-FID, carbon monoxide testing using spectrometric techniques, heavy metal analysis using inductively coupled plasma mass spectrometry, and GUS using GC-MS and LC-MS/MS to confirm all suspected positive results. GUS depends on the case, and target drugs and their metabolites in specimens of interest, which include but are not limited to opiates, opioids, amphetamines, cocaine, benzodiazepines, barbiturates, antipsychotics, cannabinoids, and their metabolites, were identified using adapted LC-MS/MS methods as previously reported [23–25], while GUS for non-target drugs was performed using GC-MS [26,27].

2.5. Statistical Analysis

Useful statistical data are reported in terms of the frequency, percentage, mean, median, and range when applicable. The data were calculated using Statistical Packages for Software Sciences (SPSS) version 28.0.1.1 (Armonk, New York, IBM Corporation) and Microsoft Excel version 16.66.1 (Microsoft, Redmond, WA, USA). Descriptive statistics were completed, and continuous data were presented as median, minimum, and maximum. Definite data were displayed as frequency and percentage. A Mann-Whitney U test was employed to estimate variations between groups. Spearman's correlation test (R) was utilized to compare variables. A p-value <0.05 was considered statistically significant.

2.6. Method Validation

The method in the current investigation was validated according to ANSI/ASB standards [22] and other published method validation protocols [28,29]. Two different LC-MS/MS methods were fully validated using the BNaF, urine, vitreous humor, and bile samples before being employed in the current investigative analysis. Complete method validation using blood and other specimens has been published previously [20,25]. Negative human postmortem specimens that were confirmed to be drug-free were utilized for calibration and quality control. Over the 10-year study period, the method parameters were re-optimized and re-validated when needed as part of the quality control and policy and procedure protocol updates, as required by the JPCC. Calibration curves of the matrices of interest were prepared for each new batch of samples according to the sample type (each calibrator was run in duplicate). Linear dynamic range (LDR) was chosen as the quantitative analysis method according to previous reports [20], using a 10-point calibration curve (1000, 500, 250, 100, 50, 25, 10, 5, 1, and 0.5 ng/mL). For each matrix of interest, three positive quality control (QC) standards were established at low, medium, and high analyte concentrations (25 ng/mL, 100 ng/mL, and 800 ng/mL, respectively), which were analyzed on the same day, and this was repeated on five consecutive days (five replicates for each concentration) to investigate the within-run and between-run precision.

Heroin biomarkers are not stable, which leads to a decrease in the concentration of these biomarkers in tested specimens that are not stored properly; therefore, a sensitive method is required to measure these biomarkers. The stability of these heroin biomarkers is a well-known issue that must be considered during sample processing, namely, during sample storage, preparation, and analysis in an autosampler. Therefore, all specimens were immediately frozen, thawed before extraction, and then immediately refrozen after sampling. The stability of these heroin biomarkers was investigated in an autosampler using three controls that were previously used in precision studies, and they were reanalyzed after 24 h, 48 h, and one week.

The most important feature of such analysis methods is to investigate the limit of detection (LOD) in the proposed matrix of interest and the workable lower limit of quantification (LOQ) that can be utilized to quantify these unstable analytes at very low concentrations (≤ 1 ng/mL). Elevated morphine concentrations in urine and bile were used as the upper limit of quantification (ULOQ) and assessed for all heroin-related analytes. The sensitivity analysis was performed in accordance with the ANSI/ASB method validation guidelines [22].

In each batch of samples, negative blank samples from different matrices were included without any standards or internal standards. Negative blank samples with internal standards were only used to investigate method selectivity, and negative blank samples were run following the calibrator with the highest concentration to investigate any carryover. Matrix effects were investigated using post-extraction addition as reported by Matuszewski et al. [28]. Six different autopsy specimens were analyzed for each matrix of interest using the optimized method. These matrices were negative, and three concentrations, such as those used for precision and accuracy studies, were analyzed (each concentration was repeated five times). The same approach was used to calculate extraction recoveries for these different matrix sources, while standards were added before extraction and internal standards were added post-extraction for the recovery experiment. Matrix effects were obtained by comparison with neat standards prepared in the initial mobile phase, and the extraction recovery value was assessed via comparison with the matrix effect results as described by Matuszewski et al. [28].

3. Results

3.1. Method Validation

The validated analysis method was acceptable (Table S1), and the sensitivity of the proposed method for detecting incredibly low concentrations of heroin biomarkers and higher concentrations of morphine in urine and bile had an LOQ of 1 ng/mL for all analytes. As indicated in Table S1, the autosampler was set to 4 °C during the stability experiments, which showed that the three controls were stable up to one week, with concentrations of analytes of interest expressed as percentages to their target concentration, which were within ±10%. As most heroin users are known to be polydrug users, the ability of the method to distinguish between analytes of interest and other co-ingested drugs is crucial, especially when opioids with similar drug chemistry can be used. Peaks were not observed in the chromatogram following the injection of blank samples alone, internal standards, or standards of the analytes of interest. Similar results were obtained when only internal standards were injected and no response to heroin biomarkers, morphine, or codeine was observed. This confirmed that both the standards and the internal standards were pure.

Linearity was accepted, with coefficients of determination greater than 0.99 for 6-MAM, 6-AC, morphine, and codeine in multiple body fluid samples. The LOD values were estimated from ten different calibration curves and ranged between 0.2 and 0.4 ng/g, while the LOQ was evaluated by spiking with 1 ng/mL of each analyte of interest, and the results were calculated using freshly prepared calibration curves for all analytes of interest in different matrices of interest. The precision, accuracy, dilution, and autosampler stability results were all within 15% of the nominal value, thus confirming that the method is suitable for the quantification of target analytes in the matrices of interest. In addition, carryover contamination from the previous positive control test was not detected.

3.2. Case Samples

3.2.1. Demographic Profile

The number of heroin-related deaths in the city of Jeddah within the study period represents 2% of the total number of postmortem cases received by the JPCC between 2008 and 2018 (Figure 1). Although the Jeddah population has increased in recent years, the number of heroin-related fatalities has remained unchanged, with a median of 9 cases per year (ranging 4–15 cases/year). Almost 70% of the heroin-related deaths occurred among Saudi citizens, while 30% occurred among other nationalities. In addition, 64% of the deceased were unemployed and supported by their families. As indicated in Figure 2 and Table S2, the median BNaF morphine concentration was 282 ng/mL (n = 85; range, 23–4400 ng/mL); the highest median BNaF morphine concentration occurred in 2012 (470 ng/mL), while the lowest median concentration occurred in 2008 (141 ng/mL).

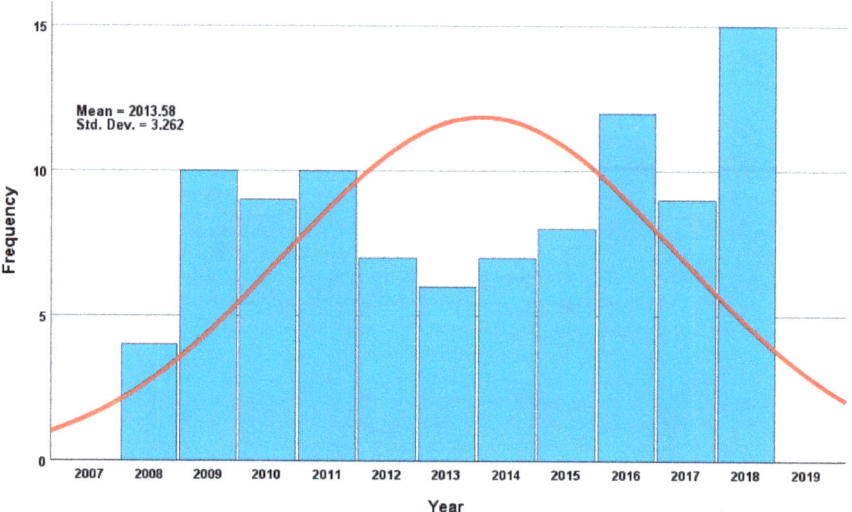

Figure 1. The total number of heroin-related deaths cases over the 10-year period in Jeddah, Saudi Arabia (2008–2018).

3.2.2. Age Groups and Analyte Concentrations

The mean age of the patients was 38 ± 12 years (range, 16–70 years; males, 98%). The 21–30 age group had the highest number of deaths, with almost 33% of the total cases (n = 32 cases), followed by the 31–40 age group (n = 26 cases, 27%), while the 10–20 age group had the lowest number of heroin-related death cases (n = 4 cases, 4%; Figure 3 and Table S3). Notably, a gradual increase in the median blood morphine concentration occurred from the youngest to the oldest age groups, with a median of 190 ng/mL in the 10–20 group and 302 ng/mL in the 51–70 group. This was also observed for morphine in the vitreous humor; in relation to age, the 6-MAM median concentration showed the same trend as morphine. 6-MAM was not detected in 75% of the cases in the 10–20 year age group, whereas it was present in 40% in the 61–70 year age group and at concentrations (BNaF median, 21 ng/mL; vitreous humor median, 52 ng/mL). This can be understood by the increase in tolerance that occurred as the duration of heroin addiction increased. Therefore, 6-MAM was more likely to be detected in the older age groups than the younger age groups. In contrast, 6-MAM was higher in the biliary specimens of the youngest age groups, as indicated in Figure 3.

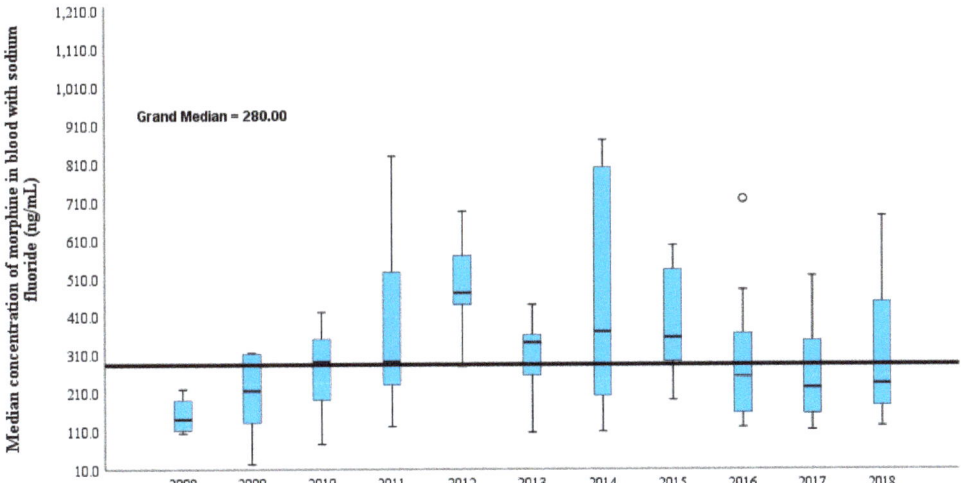

Figure 2. Variation in median concentration of morphine in blood with sodium fluoride in heroin-related deaths cases over a 10-year period. The horizontal boxes correspond to the median concentration ratio, and the box lengths correspond to the 25–75th percentile. The whiskers correspond to the smallest and largest value within 1.5 times the interquartile range, and circles (outlier) symbolize values exceeding at least 1.5 times the interquartile range and extremes (asterisks) correspond to values exceeding at least 3.0 times the interquartile range.

In the current investigation, 6-AC was more likely to be detected in the middle-aged groups and was detected in most urine samples in all age groups in this study. This finding indicates that urine is the best choice matrix for 6-AC analysis in both antemortem and postmortem samples [17,30,31]. In relation to age, the codeine concentration in the blood was slightly higher in the older age groups.

3.2.3. PMI and Analyte Concentrations

The majority of cases had a PMI within 24 h (51% of total cases), which led to the identification of both heroin biomarkers when the blood was fresh and putrefaction was not observed. The median concentrations of 6-MAM and 6-AC in cases with a PMI within 24 h were 16 and 2 ng/mL, 22 and 3 ng/mL, 324 and 35 ng/mL, and 12 and 4 ng/mL in the BNaF, vitreous humor, urine, and bile samples, respectively (Table S4). 6-AC was present in the blood at extremely low concentrations in cases where the PMI was less than 48 h, and no 6-AC was detected in any BNaF cases when the PMI was greater than 48 h, although most cases were stored properly following death. In contrast, 6-AC was still detected in the urine samples from all PMI groups (Figure 4). As expected, the median morphine concentration in BNaF increased with longer PMIs. The lowest median morphine concentration (263 ng/mL) was observed at a PMI of 24 h, and the highest concentration (380 ng/mL) was observed at a PMI ranging from 121–240 h (Figure S1).

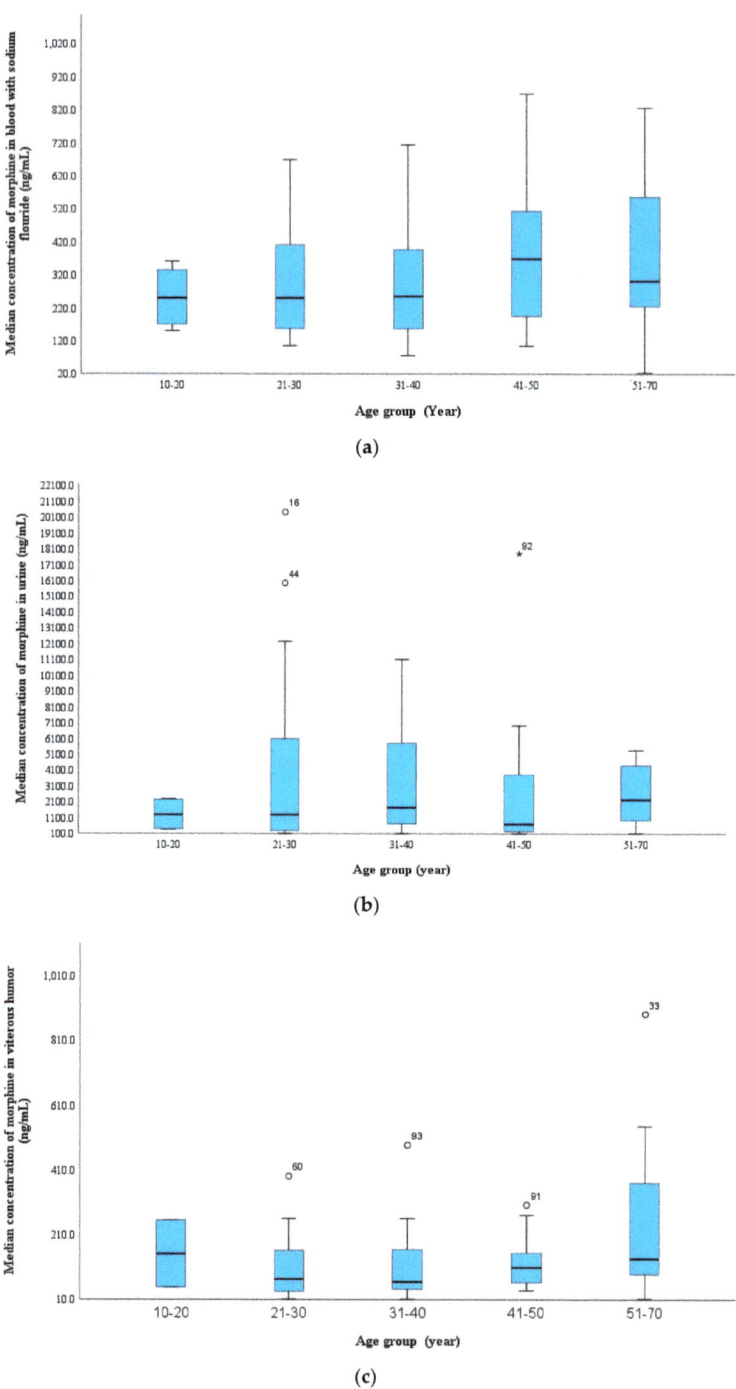

Figure 3. *Cont.*

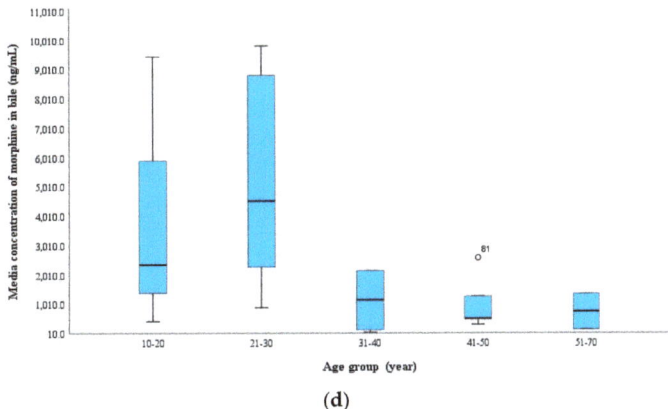

(d)

Figure 3. Variation of morphine concentration in the 97 heroin-related fatality cases according to age group (**a**) blood with sodium fluoride (ng/mL), (**b**) urine (ng/mL), (**c**) vitreous humor and (**d**) bile. The whiskers correspond to the smallest and largest value within 1.5 times the interquartile range, and circles (outlier) symbolize values exceeding at least 1.5 times the interquartile range and extremes (asterisks) correspond to values exceeding at least 3.0 times the interquartile range (this description is applied to the remaining box-plot figures).

In the current study, both biomarkers were detected in the vitreous humor in two cases with a PMI longer than 10 days, whereas 6-MAM was negative in the BNaF samples, which indicates that the role of PMIs on heroin biomarkers can be minimized if samples are stored correctly following autopsy and if the vitreous humor is the sample of choice for heroin-related fatality investigations. Figure S2 shows the distribution of 6-MAM in BNaF and vitreous humor samples among PMI groups in the current study.

3.2.4. Mode of Death

In the current study, heroin alone contributed to death in 68% of the studied cases, whereas intoxication with other co-ingested substances contributed to 32% (Table 2). A higher median morphine concentration (310 ng/mL) was observed in the heroin-only cause of death cases than in the polydrug intoxication group (250 ng/mL). The median 6-MAM concentration was similar between these two groups, whereas the median 6-AC concentration in the heroin-alone cases was higher (2.5-fold) than that in the polydrug intoxication group. No difference was observed between the codeine concentrations in the two groups.

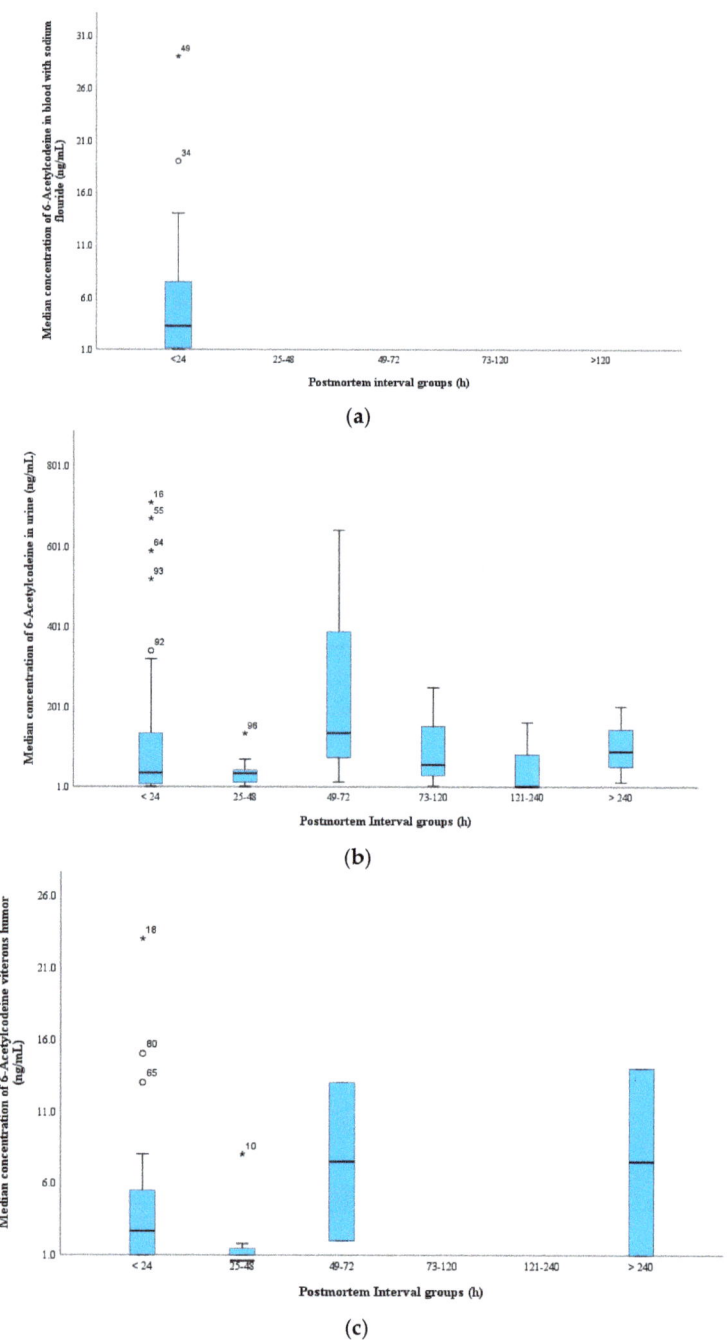

Figure 4. *Cont.*

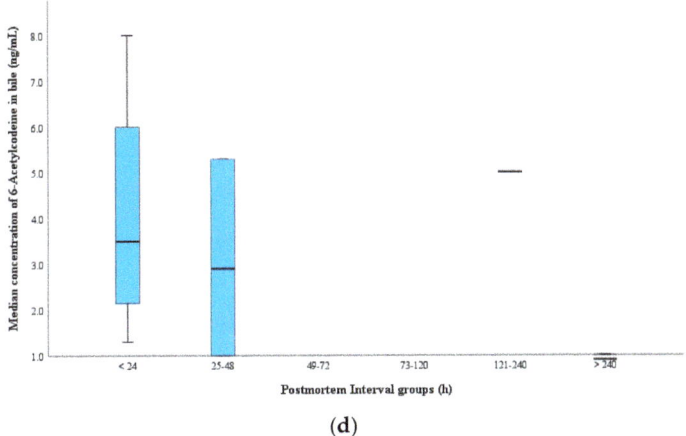

(d)

Figure 4. Distribution of 6-AC in the 97 heroin-related fatality cases according to postmortem interval time group (**a**) blood with sodium fluoride (ng/mL), (**b**) urine (ng/mL), (**c**) vitreous humor and (**d**) bile. The whiskers correspond to the smallest and largest value within 1.5 times the interquartile range, and circles (outlier) symbolize values exceeding at least 1.5 times the interquartile range and extremes (asterisks) correspond to values exceeding at least 3.0 times the interquartile range (this description is applied to the remaining box-plot figures).

Table 2. Heroin biomarkers, morphine, and codeine concentration in relation to cause of death in the current study.

		Cause of Deaths							
		Heroin Only				Poly Drug Intoxication			
	Total case number	66				31			
		N	Med	Min	Max	N	Med	Min	Max
Specimens	Analytes [&]		ng/mL				ng/mL		
Blood with Sodium Fluoride	6-MAM	36	10	1	420	14	10	Tr	100
	6-AC	11	5	Tr	30	9	2	Tr	10
	Morphine	57	310	100	4400	27	250	23	670
	Codeine	57	20	4	140	27	20	3	110
Urine	6-MAM	46	330	1	18,900	28	320	1	4600
	6-AC	30	40	1	670	20	40	1	710
	Morphine	46	1340	90	50,400	2	1850	10	20,400
	Codeine	43	210	5	12,110	27	170	3	1210
Vitreous Humor	6-MAM	45	30	1	240	25	20	1	210
	6-AC	18	2	Tr	10	17	2	Tr	20
	Morphine	45	90	10	890	26	90	10	490
	Codeine	44	10	3	140	25	10	1	70
Bile	6-MAM	9	10	1	160	8	10	2	40
	6-AC	3	5	1	10	5	3	1	5
	Morphine	18	2400	40	41,100	10	1700	300	4
	Codeine	15	20	5	230	10	40	10	120

[&] Analytes: 6-monoacetylmorphine (6-MAM), 6-acetylcodeine (6-AC). N: number of cases; Med: Median; Min: Minimum; Max: Maximum; Tr: Trace concentration.

These findings indicate that the morphine concentration in heroin-related fatalities showing the presence of other CNS drugs is often lower than that in heroin-alone cases. The significant role of the PMI in cases of heroin metabolites is well known, and the tolerance and health status of the deceased contribute to this finding. Similar trends were observed among the various specimens, with slightly higher median concentrations in the urine and bile. Moreover, a polydrug intoxication case showed a slightly higher morphine concentration in the vitreous humor than that with heroin alone.

The most frequently detected drugs, regardless of the cause of death, were methamphetamine, cannabis, amphetamine, alprazolam, cocaine, and ethanol. Thirty-eight cases only showed heroin metabolites. A higher median morphine concentration was measured in only heroin cases compared to those in which heroin was the sole cause of death despite the presence of another drug, such as amphetamine or cannabis (370 ng/mL vs. 310 ng/mL). Similarly, the median morphine concentration (312 ng/mL) decreased when one extra drug was used, and it was further decreased (191 and 198 ng/mL) when two and four extra drugs were co-ingested, respectively.

Notably, methamphetamine was co-ingested with heroin in twenty-three cases (BNaF median morphine concentration, 284 ng/mL). The median morphine concentration for most co-ingested drugs was often higher than 200 ng/mL. A reduction in the median morphine concentration (BNaF, 154 ng/mL) occurred when heroin was used in combination with cocaine.

3.2.5. Time Span between Heroin Intake and Death

In this study, 61% and 24% of the cases were rapid and delayed deaths, respectively, and 15% had an undetermined time of death. This was either because of a lack of information caused by the deceased dying without a witness or because the bodies were moved after death to a deserted area where the bodies began to decompose and thus did not show signs of heroin use, such as injection marks (Table 3 and Figure 5). In these cases, both heroin biomarkers tested negative in the BNaF samples. Although a higher PMI was detected in these cases, heroin biomarkers were detected in alternative body fluids, and all urine samples tested positive for 6-MAM.

Table 3. Heroin biomarkers, morphine, and codeine concentration in relation to survival time following heroin administered in the current study.

Specimens	Analytes &		Rapid Deaths				Delayed Death				Unknown		
	Total case number		69				19				9		
		$N^\#$	Median	Minimum	Maximum	N	Median	Minimum	Maximum	N	Median	Minimum	Maximum
Blood with Sodium Fluoride	6-MAM	48	10	Tr	420	0				0			
	6-AC	19	3	Tr *	30	0				0			
	MOR	66	310	80.0	4400	14	210	23.0	715	4	317	310.0	439
	COD	66	20	3.0	140	14	10	3.0	40	4	30	4.0	60
Urine	6-MAM	54	380	1.0	18,876	14	380	10.0	820	6	50	1.0	130
	6-AC	37	40	1.0	710	12	10	1.0	320	0			
	MOR	54	2100	14.0	50,401	14	1300	244.0	11,100	6	550	120.0	11,700
	COD	51	210	3.0	12,110	13	90	3.0	630	6	20	5.0	660
Vitreous Humor	6-MAM	50	40	1.3	240	18	10	3.0	40	2	n.a.	1.0	13
	6-AC	25	3	Tr	20	9	1	Tr	14	1	n.a.	1.0	1
	MOR	51	90	10.0	900	18	60	10.0	270	2	n.a	11.0	90
	COD	50	10	1.0	140	17	10	3.0	70	2	n.a.	2.0	10

Table 3. Cont.

		Survival Time											
		Rapid Deaths				Delayed Death				Unknown			
Bile	6-MAM	10	10	2.0	160	4	10	10.0	40	3	10	2.0	40
	6-AC	4	2	Tr	5	3	5	4.0	10	1	n.a	1.0	1
	MOR	17	2200	30.0	41,100	6	2800	40.0	9,400	4	1520	410.0	41,100
	COD	16	30	5.0	190	5	40	Tr	230	4	40	10.0	170

& Analytes: 6-monoacetylmorphine (6-MAM), 6-acetylcodeine (6-AC); MOR: morphine; COD: codeine.
# N: number of cases; * Tr: Trace concentration.

This suggests that either the undetermined cases died immediately after heroin was administered and the environmental surroundings allowed for the hydrolysis of 6-MAM to morphine or that a delayed death occurred, which allowed morphine glucuronide to deconjugate to free morphine due to the long PMI before sampling. In contrast, lower median morphine concentrations were observed in the delayed death group (median BNaF = 210 ng/mL) than the rapid death group.

In all groups, the median morphine concentration was much lower in the vitreous humor than the blood. This indicates that some of the heroin biomarkers were converted to their metabolites in the blood but were stable in the vitreous humor after death. Nevertheless, the vitreous humor results should be interpreted with caution because a certain amount of morphine is associated with accumulation from the use of old doses by chronic heroin users. Interestingly, 6-MAM levels were higher for the rapid death cases (36 ng/mL) than the delayed death cases (14 ng/mL) and undetermined death cases (7 ng/mL). This can be explained by many factors, including the longer PMI in delayed deaths, putrefaction effects, and body storage effects, especially when the time of death is unknown. These conditions led to a decrease in the 6-MAM concentration in the vitreous humor. This highlights the importance of testing the vitreous humor in cases of longer PMIs and negative 6-MAM in the blood.

Morphine levels in bile were primarily detected in chronic heroin users, which limits the use of these values in distinguishing between rapid and delayed deaths. 6-MAM in bile was detected in 10 of 17 rapid deaths, 3 of 6 delayed deaths, and not detected of 4 undermined cases. Urine is most likely to be positive for heroin biomarkers and their metabolites in these types of deaths. In this study, the free morphine concentration was high for rapid deaths (2100 ng/mL) compared to that for delayed deaths (1300 ng/mL) and undetermined cases (550 ng/mL). An almost 4-fold higher median concentration of 6-AC in urine was observed for rapid death (40 ng/mL) compared with delayed death (10 ng/mL). Moreover, the median codeine concentration was higher in the unknown group (30 ng/mL) than in the rapid (20 ng/mL) and delayed groups (10 ng/mL). Codeine forms quickly after heroin ingestion as a product of 6-AC degradation. Most codeine is metabolized to codeine-6-glucuronide, while some is metabolized to morphine.

3.2.6. Manner of Death

In the current study, 76% of the total cases were ascribed to accidental death, and they had a median age, median BNaF morphine concentration, and PMI of 38 years, 280 ng/mL, and 24 h, respectively. Nevertheless, most heroin abusers in Saudi Arabia used drugs in private or remote areas, such as deserted areas and open land outside the city. In the case of overdoses, deceased bodies left behind without witnesses complicated the identification of the mode of death, especially if the bodies were heavily putrefied.

Information about intentional overdoses was available for seven heroin-related fatalities. Four of these individuals died at home, and two died outdoors while accompanied by a friend. These cases had a median BNaF morphine concentration of 480 ng/mL, a PMI of 24 h, and an age of 48. The highest levels of vitreous humor and morphine were detected in suicide cases (150 ng/m).

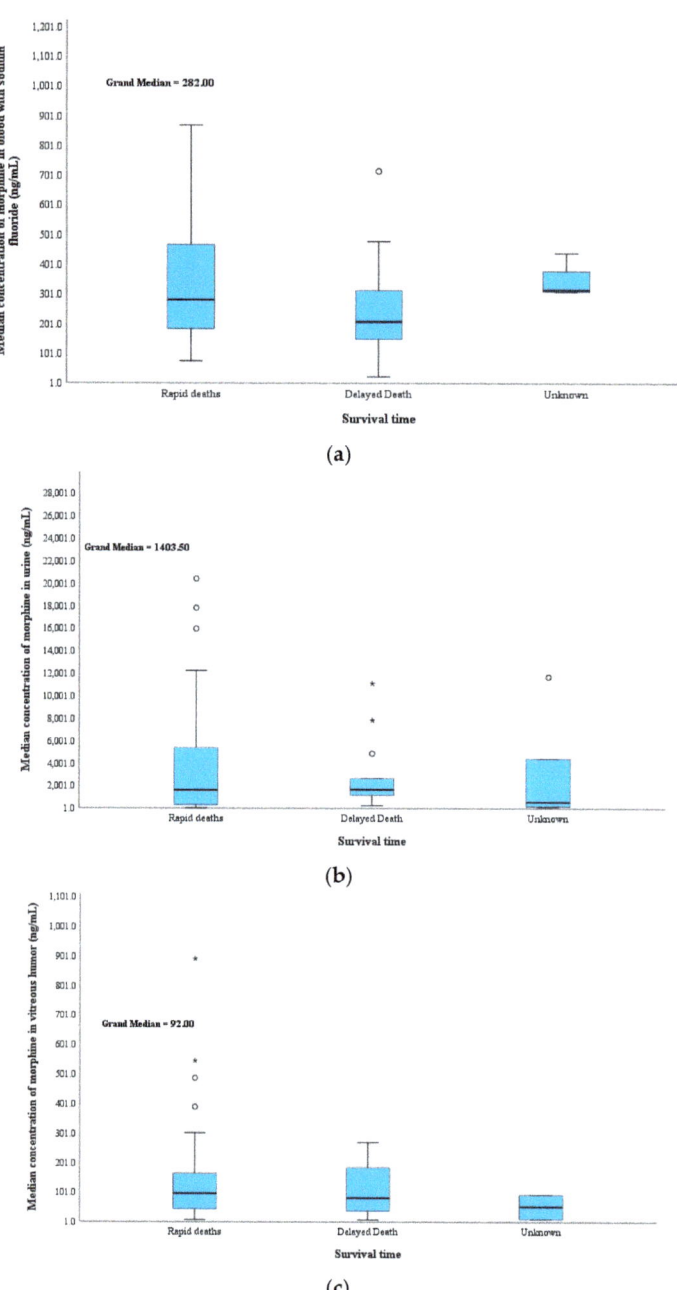

Figure 5. *Cont.*

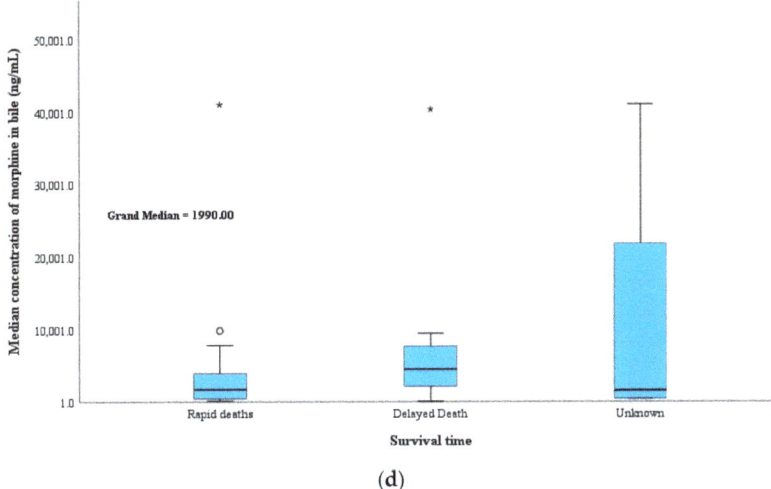

(d)

Figure 5. Variation of median morphine concentration in the 97 heroin-related fatalities cases according to survival time before death; (**a**) blood with sodium fluoride (ng/mL), (**b**) urine (ng/mL), (**c**) vitreous humor and (**d**) bile. The whiskers correspond to the smallest and largest value within 1.5 times the interquartile range, and circles (outlier) symbolize values exceeding at least 1.5 times the interquartile range and extremes (asterisks) correspond to values exceeding at least 3.0 times the interquartile range (this description is applied to the remaining box-plot figures).

In five cases, the mode of death was identified as homicide, and they presented a median BNaF morphine concentration of 180 ng/mL, a PMI of 24 h, and an age of 22. Notably, most cases were discovered outdoors.

The data in Table 4 clearly show that heroin biomarkers were higher in suicides, which had median concentrations of 210 ng/mL for 6-MAM. The role of multiple specimens was crucial for the undetected modes of death because few blood specimens were available for testing. The detection of heroin biomarkers facilitates the source of opioid identification and survival time. In some cases, although syringes and heroin bags were found at the scene, the blood samples were negative for heroin biomarkers. No difference in codeine concentrations was observed according to the mode of death. The manner of deaths was not determined in the last 11 cases.

Table 4. Heroin biomarkers, morphine, and codeine concentration in relation to manner of death in the current study.

		Manner of Deaths															
		Accidental				Suicidal				Homicidal				Undetermined			
Total Case Number		74				7				5				11			
Specimens	Analytes &	N#	Median	Minimum	Maximum	N	Median	Minimum	Maximum	N	Median	Minimum	Maximum	N	Median	Minimum	Maximum
				ng/mL				ng/mL				ng/mL				ng/mL	
Blood with Sodium Fluoride	6-MAM	39	10	Tr*	150	6	210	5.0	420	2	6	2.0	10	3	3	1.0	20
	6-AC	15	2	Tr	10	5	10	4.0	30	0				0			
	MOR	67	280	20.0	830	7	480	220.0	4400	3	180	150.0	870	7	210	120.0	720
	COD	67	20	3.0	110	7	30	5.0	140	3	10	4.0	50	7	10	4.0	40
Urine	6-MAM	57	310	1.0	4600	6	810	30.0	18,900	5	480	54.0	2520	6	540	40.0	1580
	6-AC	36	36	1.0	710	5	40	13.0	670	4	40	1.0	250	5	10	1.0	160
	MOR	57	1330	10.0	20,400	6	3630	100.0	50,400	5	2100	1240.0	5350	6	990	190.0	4110
	COD	54	140	3.0	1300	6	240	5.0	12,110	4	540	170.0	1210	6	150	10.0	2100
Vitreous Humor	6-MAM	57	20	1.0	200	5	210	60.0	240	3	20	3.0	30	5	20	1.0	50
	6-AC	28	2	Tr	20	5	3	1.0	10	1	10	10.0	10	1	1	1.0	1
	MOR	57	80	10.0	890	5	150	40.0	550	3	50	40.0	150	6	120	40.0	300
	COD	55	10	1.0	140	5	20	10.0	30	3	10	10.0	10	6	10	3.0	20
Bile	6-MAM	9	10	2.0	40	1	10	10.0	10	2	30	10.0	40	5	2	1.0	160
	6-AC	5	3	1.0	5	0				2	4	Tr	10	1	5	5.0	5
	MOR	16	2100	40.0	41,100	2	310	130.0	490	3	1350	1260.0	9440	7	2807	120.0	41,100
	COD	13	40	10.0	170	2	20	10.0	20	3	70	5.0	230	7	10	10	190

& Analytes: 6-monoacetylmorphine (6-MAM), 6-acetylcodeine (6-AC); MOR: morphine; COD: codeine. # N: number of cases; * Tr: Trace concentration.

3.2.7. Route of Administration

Table 5 demonstrates that heroin injection was the main route of administration in the current investigation, followed by sniffing. The route of administration was unknown in 16 of cases, with most involving decomposed bodies. Syringes were found at the scene in 36% of the studied cases. Needle marks were identified in 65% of the total cases, whereas heroin powder was found in 18% of the total cases. Heroin was sniffed in only 9% of cases, which indicates that injection is the main route of heroin administration in Saudi Arabia.

Table 5. Comparison of different routes of administration on heroin biomarkers, morphine, and codeine concentrations in the 97 heroin-related fatalities cases in Jeddah, Saudi Arabia between 2008–2018.

		Route of Administration											
		Injection				Sniffing				Unknown			
	Total Case Number	72				9				16			
Specimens	Analytes &	N #	Median	Minimum	Maximum	N	Median	Minimum	Maximum	N	Median	Minimum	Maximum
Blood with Sodium Fluoride	6-MAM	41	10	1.0	420	5	4	Tr	10	4	5	1.3	20
	6-Ac	17	4	Tr *	30	3	3	Tr	10	0			
	Morphine	63	310	20.0	4400	8	150	75.0	360	13	220	120.0	720
	Codeine	63	20	3.0	140	8	10	3.0	40	13	20	10.0	70
Urine	6-MAM	53	470	1.0	18,900	9	280	20.0	480	12	75	1.0	2520
	6-Ac	36	40	1.0	710	7	20	1.0	40	7	10	1.0	250
	Morphine	53	2650	10.0	50,400	9	1330	20.0	11,700	12	310	90.0	5350
	Codeine	52	220	3.0	12,110	7	140	3.0	660	11	20	5.0	1210
Vitreous Humor	6-MAM	53	25	3.0	240	9	20	3.4	125	8	30	1.0	80
	6-Ac	27	2	Tr	20	6	4	1.0	20	2	10	1.0	10
	Morphine	53	90	10.0	890	9	90	10.0	260	9	120	11.0	300
	Codeine	52	10	1.0	140	9	10	3.0	20	8	10	200	30
Bile	6-MAM	8	10	2.0	40	6	10	10.0	40	3	10	1.0	160
	6-Ac	2	3	1.0	5	5	4	1.0	10	1	1	1.0	1
	Morphine	16	1590	130.0	41,100	6	4180	1510.0	9440	6	1060	40.0	403400
	Codeine	15	30	5.0	170	6	50	20.0	230	4	20	10	190

& Analytes: 6-monoacetylmorphine (6-MAM), 6-acetylcodeine (6-AC); MOR: morphine; COD: codeine. # N: number of cases; * Tr: Trace concentration.

Table 6 indicates that the median morphine BNaF concentration when the drug was administered via injection was 300 ng/mL, followed by sniffing at 150 ng/mL and an unknown route of administration at 220 ng/mL (Table 5). The highest BNaF morphine concentrations (340 ng/mL and 310 ng/mL) were observed when heroin powder and syringes were found near the deceased, respectively. In cases where both syringes and heroin powder were discovered, the median BNaF morphine concentration was 400 ng/mL. No differences were observed in the median vitreous humor concentration among the three routes of administration, with a median of 90–120 ng/mL in all groups. The heroin powder group showed a slightly higher morphine vitreous humor concentration, followed by cases with syringes and heroin bags at 160 ng/mL and 140 ng/mL, respectively (Table S5). In contrast, the median urine morphine concentration was higher in cases of injected heroin (2400 ng/mL) than in the sniffing heroin group (1400 ng/mL). The median bile morphine concentration was almost double in the sniffing group (4200 ng/mL) than in the injection group (1600 ng/mL).

Table 6. Location of deaths and state of deceased body at autopsy in the 97 heroin-related fatalities cases in Jeddah, Saudi Arabia between 2008–2018.

			Location of Death									Putrefaction							
			Indoor				Outdoor				Non-Putrefied				Partial Putrefied				Heavy Putrefied
Total Case Number			36				61				76				13				8
	Analytes &	N #	Median	Minimum	Maximum	N	Median	Minimum	Maximum	N	Median	Minimum	Maximum	N	Median	Minimum	Maximum	N	Median	Minimum	Maximum	N
Blood with Sodium Fluoride	6-MAM	21	10	Tr*	420	29	10	1.0	150	46	10	Tr	420	2	10	1.0	10	2	10	3.0	20
	6-AC	9	4	Tr	30	11	2	Tr	10	20	3	Tr	30	0							
	MOR	33	320	20.0	4400	51	240	100.0	830	68	270	20.0	4400	10	320	121.0	725	6	370	200.0	720
	COD	33	20	3.0	140	51	20	3.0	110	68	20	3.0	140	10	20	3.0	60	6	20	4.0	70
Urine	6-MAM	30	310	10.0	18,900	44	360	1.0	4600	60	320	1.0	18,900	8	340	1.0	2520	6	540	130.0	1580
	6-AC	17	30	3.0	670	33	40	1.0	710	39	35	Tr	710	6	50	1.0	250	5	10	2.0	160
	MOR	30	1090	100.0	42,300	44	2030	10.0	50,400	60	1850	10.0	42,300	8	710	122.0	50,400	6	1140	520.0	4110
	COD	28	180	5.0	12,110	42	210	3.0	2100	56	200	3.0	12,110	8	50	3.0	1590	6	130	10.0	2100
Vitreous Humor	6-MAM	27	40	10.0	240	43	20	1.0	215	60	20	1.0	240	6	40	1.0	220	4	25	20.0	30
	6-AC	12	3	Tr	20	23	1	Tr	15	32	2	Tr	20	2	10	1.0	10	1	1	1.0	1
	MOR	27	100	10.0	490	44	80	10.0	890	60	70	10.0	890	6	220	11.0	550	5	140	40.0	300
	COD	26	20	3.0	70	43	10	1.0	140	58	10	1.0	140	6	15	2.0	30	5	10	3.0	10
Bile	6-MAM	9	10	2.0	40	8	10	1.0	160	12	10	1.0	160	3	10	2.0	40	2	10	2.0	10
	6-AC	3	1	1.0	3	5	5	1.0	10	6	2	Tr	10	1	4	4.0	4	1	5	5.0	5
	MOR	14	1075	40.0	7800	14	3520	120.0	41,100	21	1830	120.0	41,100	4	1520	40.0	4470	3	2150	490.0	40,400
	COD	12	20	5.0	120	13	70	10	230	19	30	5.0	230	3	40	13.0	40	3	70	10.0	190

& Analytes: 6-monoacetylmorphine (6-MAM), 6-acetylcodeine (6-AC). # N: number of cases; * Tr: Trace concentration.

3.2.8. Location of Deaths and Putrefaction

Most heroin deaths occurred in outdoor environments (63%), with a median PMI of 48 h, whereas 37% of the patients died in a private home (Table 6), with a median PMI of 24 h. A higher median BNaF morphine level was observed in those who died indoors (320 ng/mL) than outdoors (240 ng/mL), while the level in vitreous humor was similar (100 ng/mL vs. 80 ng/mL, respectively). In contrast, the median urine and bile morphine concentrations were two- and three-fold higher among those who died outdoors than indoors, respectively.

It has been mentioned that the weather in Saudi Arabia is extremely hot most of the year, and the weather in Jeddah is known to be highly humid. Accordingly, it is well-known that putrefaction and postmortem changes would begin a few hours following death if bodies were not stored appropriately [32,33]. In cases in which heroin was injected and the person dies alone in a closed indoor area, putrefaction will occur faster owing to the combination of hot weather and high humidity in Jeddah city. Considering that most of the deceased die indoors and are discovered in a closed toilet, garage, or hidden area at home, such as the roof, this could facilitate postmortem changes, especially when deaths occur at night with no witnesses. In contrast, a deceased body on the street (outdoor) would be easily discovered unless it was moved to an empty or deserted area.

In 63 out of 97 cases (65%), police and forensic pathologist reports indicated that no witnesses observed the final moments before death (Table S5). Nine patients (11%) were transferred to the hospital; however, most patients died either at the scene before transfer to the hospital or during transfer to the hospital. Identifying the mode of death was difficult due to a lack of information and heavy decomposition of the bodies, especially for those who died outdoors, in the desert, under construction bridges, or in old buildings. In 8 of the 97 cases, the manner of death was unknown due to putrefaction, and these cases presented a median BNaF morphine concentration of 380 ng/mL, a PMI of 230 h, and an age of 40. High morphine concentrations can be explained by the administration of a high dose or due to postmortem changes after death that cause the conversion of 6-MAM and morphine conjugates to free morphine.

In this study, higher BNaF morphine concentrations were measured in patients whose deaths were pronounced at hospitals (n = 9 cases, 450 ng/mL), followed by those found in the street (n = 9 cases, 335 ng/mL), under bridges (n = 11 cases, 262 ng/mL), in cars (n = 17, 240 ng/mL), in rental flats or hotel rooms (n = 7, 237 ng/mL), and in deserted areas (n = 8 cases, 170 ng/mL). PMI, environmental conditions (location of death and weather), and patient tolerance have major effects on the detection of heroin biomarkers and metabolites. The patients who died at the hospital had a lower PMI, and their deaths were caused by an overdose of heroin alone. In contrast, among individuals who died under bridges, most cases showed putrefaction, and 6 out of 10 cases were polydrug intoxication cases. Notably, a high number of deaths occurred in cars, with 13 out of 17 cases of polydrug intoxication having a relatively low PMI (median 24 h) and 6 cases exhibiting signs of putrefaction, with two heavily putrefied. Vitreous humor and urine were available in 13 and 12 of these cases, respectively, and 6-MAM and 6-AC were detected in 6 and 9 cases, respectively. Only one case was positive for both heroin biomarkers in bile. A higher median of BNaF morphine was observed compared to vitreous humor (60 ng/mL), which suggested a shorter survival time. This was supported by the lower urine morphine concentration (860 ng/mL) and highest bile morphine concentration (9800 ng/mL), suggesting a chronic heroin user.

Twenty-one cases showed signs of putrefaction (Table 6), 60% showed partial purification, and 8 out of 21 putrefied cases showed heavy decomposition. There was no difference in age between the two groups; however, the PMIs were higher in the heavily putrefied group (heavy putrefaction: 228 h; partial putrefaction: 96 h; Table 6). 6-MAM was detected in BNaF in two cases in each group. The advantages of testing alternative specimens in determining the source of opioids have been clearly observed in these putrefaction cases because most of the alternative samples, namely urine, vitreous humor, and bile, were positive for 6-MAM. A few cases that showed partial putrefaction tested positive for 6-AC.

3.2.9. Seasonal Distribution

The seasonal distribution of heroin-related fatalities is presented in Table S6 and Figure S3. The highest proportion occurred in spring (29%), followed by summer (28%), winter (27%), and autumn (16%). The highest mortality rate occurred in July (12%), followed by April (11%). The lowest proportion of heroin fatalities (4 %) occurred in October.

3.2.10. Multiple Specimens

The median morphine concentrations in the BNaF, urine, vitreous humor, and bile samples were 280, 1400, 90, and 2200 ng/mL, respectively. Among the available BNaF, urine, vitreous humor, and bile specimens, 6-MAM was detected in 60%, 100%, 99%, and 59%, while 6-AC was detected in 24%, 68%, 50%, and 30%, respectively. The presence of sodium fluoride in the blood test tube as a preservative prevented 6-MAM from converting to morphine in most cases. Additionally, the availability of urine, bile, and vitreous humor samples provides valuable information on the opioids that have been administered. The median free morphine concentration ratios among the vitreous humor/BNaF, urine/BNaF, and bile/BNaF were 0.37-fold (n = 63), 5.6-fold (n = 64), and 7.3-fold (n = 23), respectively. In addition, free morphine/free codeine were always higher than 1, with median ratios of 13-fold (n = 84), 13-fold (n = 70), 6-fold (n = 68), and 85-fold (n = 25) for BNaF, urine, vitreous humor, and bile, respectively.

The Spearman correlation coefficient (R) was used to establish the relationship between heroin biomarkers, morphine, and codeine concentrations in various body fluids (Table S7). 6-MAM in BNaF exhibited a strong positive correlation with the analytes of interest in both the urine and vitreous humor, except for 6-MAM in BNaF vs. 6-AC in the vitreous humor. In contrast, the correlation between 6-MAM in BNaF and analytes of interest in bile was weakly positive for 6-MAM, 6-AC, and codeine but negative for morphine (non-significant p-values higher than 0.5). The correlation between the 6-AC concentration obtained from multiple biological fluids was always poor and not statistically significant, and it was not calculated for bile due to the lack of positive samples. A negative correlation was observed between 6-AC and morphine in bile and analytes of interest in the BNaF, urine, and vitreous humor samples, as shown in Table S7. The poor correlation between 6-AC in the different specimens could be explained by the low concentrations, small sample size, and instability of 6-AC in biological specimens. The 6-AC concentrations in BNaF were not significantly correlated with the analytes of interest in the urine and bile, while a significant correlation was obtained with the analytes of interest in the vitreous humor.

Good correlations were obtained between the analytes of interest detected in BNaF vs. vitreous humor, BNAF vs. urine, and vitreous humor vs. urine. The level of 6-AC seemed to be higher in the vitreous humor than the blood, which can directly reflect the anatomical location of the vitreous humor; thus, 6-AC in the vitreous humor is more stable and has a longer half-life before conversion to codeine than that in blood samples.

The bile samples showed the lowest positive results for 6-AC (eight cases) compared to 6-MAM. The 6-MAM was detected in 16 of the 27 bile samples tested in this study. Although the correlation between heroin-related compounds in BNaF and bile was weak, the correlation between these analytes in bile and their corresponding specimens in vitreous humor and urine was strong, except for the 6-AC concentration.

4. Discussion

4.1. History of Heroin Abuse

In the literature, few studies have detailed the relationship between addiction and morphine concentration. Steentoft et al. reported 245 heroin-related deaths, and all of these cases were from known heroin abusers with the exception of 13 cases [34]. Elfawal pointed out the lack of history of drug abuse in opiate overdose cases in the eastern region of Saudi Arabia [14]. In the current study, a history of heroin abuse was observed in only 24% of all cases. This indicates an improvement in healthcare reporting regarding postmortem drug abuse in Saudi Arabia, considering that the Elfawal study was conducted in 1999 [14].

4.2. Age Group and Analyte Concentrations

Heroin users often die young because of polydrug intoxication [35], and most of the deceased are male. Previous reports showed that middle-aged groups and individuals from 21–40 were most likely to be at risk of heroin intoxication, which was demonstrated in the current study based on this group accounting for 60% of the total cases. In one study from Jordan, the mean age of five cases of heroin-related death was 33 [36]. In the eastern region of Saudi Arabia, Elfawal reported that almost 60% of drug-related deaths occurred in individuals aged 20–29 years old [14]. A study from Iran reported that 34% of opioid-related fatalities occurred in individuals aged 20–29 years [37]. In Victoria, Australia, the median ages of opioid-related fatalities were 30 and 29 for males and females, respectively [38]. In Sweden, the median age of heroin-related deaths ranges from 34 to 35 in two different studies [2,39]. An older mean age of 47 has been reported for Minneapolis, MA, USA [40]

Jones and Ahlner studied 766 postmortem heroin-related deaths and 124 traffic antemortem cases related to heroin use and found no correlation between the concentration of free morphine and the age of heroin users (r = 009, $p > 0.05$) [2]. These findings were consistent with those reported by Darke et al. [41]. It is believed that older heroin users likely received higher doses, developed tolerance, and were less likely to change their drug use practices. In the present study, a higher median morphine concentration in the blood was observed in individuals older than 40 compared to those younger than 40, which may be related to the increased tolerance to heroin in long-term abuse cases. A higher 6-MAM level was detected in the blood of the older age group (the highest 6-MAM median blood concentration (250 ng/mL) was found in the 61–70-year age group), while 6-AC was found at low concentrations in all age groups.

The level of codeine was low in all age groups (median, 20–35 ng/mL), which could be explained by the fact that 6-AC is metabolized to codeine and codeine-6-glucuronide (C6G) faster than to other compounds. A recently published study demonstrated that C6G was not detected in blood samples obtained from authentic postmortem cases following heroin intake, while codeine was [42]. In another study, codeine was always higher than C6G in autopsy blood samples from heroin- and codeine-related fatalities [19]. Thus, reporting the free codeine concentrations in the blood is accurate and less laborious. In contrast, C6G was frequently present at a much higher concentration than codeine in many cases attributed to codeine intoxication [43].

4.3. PMI and Analytes Concentration

Skopp concluded that the PMI competes with the postmortem redistribution phenomenon (PMR) [44], and they indicated that postmortem changes that occur between death and the discovery of the body include degradation and the formation of drugs or new products. These changes may occur before autopsy and during sample transfer and storage, which is consistent with the many cases of ethanol synthesis after death, for example. Changes that occur during the PMI period and the stability of heroin biomarkers have been well addressed in the literature and can be investigated by assessing the conditions surrounding the cases under investigation, such as the condition of the body after putrefaction has started. A longer PMI can decrease and increase the amounts of heroin biomarkers and their metabolites, respectively, and the presence of these heroin biomarkers cannot be detected with a longer PMI. However, Gerostamoulos and Drummer [45] investigated the influence of PMR on heroin-related fatalities (n = 40, mean PMI = 59 h) and did not observe significant changes in morphine and its metabolite concentrations between antemortem and postmortem samples. This observation was supported by the work of Logan and Smirnow, who also found no significant difference in free morphine concentrations obtained from different anatomical sites (n = 32 cases) [46]. In 19 cases related to codeine intoxication, they found that the PMI did not have a significant effect on the production, formation, or redistribution of codeine-related metabolites, including morphine and its metabolites [43].

Fugelstad et al. studied the effects of postmortem changes on heroin-related fatalities and concluded that the concentration detected at autopsy was the same as that at the time of death [39]. In contrast, Sawyer and Forney studied the effect of different PMIs on the concentration of morphine in rats and found that the morphine metabolites increased by almost 300% [47]. This increase may be due to the fast release of fluids from tissues following death in small animals, which leads to increased morphine concentrations in postmortem body fluids [45,46]. Although morphine concentrations differed depending on the site of collection, such as cardiac blood and femoral blood, this can be due to the incomplete distribution of the drug after death and mostly represents anatomical site-to-site differences, which should be considered when interpreting heroin-related fatalities [4,45,48].

PMR has been debated scientifically, especially for postmortem blood morphine concentrations following heroin-related deaths. Maskell et al. suggested the use of vitreous fluid to verify heroin use because minimal morphine change was detected in their study [49]. An increase in free morphine after death can be expected due to the conversion of 6-MAM to morphine; in some cases, morphine-conjugated degradation can be expected, especially during the PMI period [2,50,51]. Including multiple specimens is crucial for identifying the source of the opiates used. In the case of vitreous humor, this study showed that 6-MAM is higher than BNaF in this fluid and free morphine is lower than BNaF. Similar observations were reported by Scott and Oliver [52] and Rees et al. [51]. Different results have been obtained for urine samples because low free morphine concentrations should be expected due to morphine-conjugated formation before excretion into urine [53,54]. Heroin biomarkers were more stable in vitreous fluid than in blood [55], which is supported by the detection of high 6-MAM in vitreous humor in cases with a longer PMI, whereas 6-MAM was negative or found at a low level in BNaF samples. The probability of obtaining a vitreous humor specimen for testing decreases with an increase in the time between death and body discovery. In addition, longer PMIs decreased the likelihood of obtaining such specimens unless the body was stored properly immediately after death [33]. The combination of BNaF and vitreous fluids or BNaF and urine analysis are crucial tools for identifying the source of morphine in postmortem cases with a PMI greater than 48 h. Bile is a unique matrix for assessing the chronic use of drugs [20], and it was tested in only 27 cases in the current investigation. Interestingly, both heroin biomarkers were detected in all PMI period groups; however, due to the small sample size in the long PMI groups, we could not examine the correlation between BNaF and bile when assessing heroin-related deaths. However, the presence of heroin biomarkers might be a potential indicator of a recent, rapid overdose of heroin, regardless of the PMI period after death. Codeine is formed by 6-AC degradation, and most of the 6-AC is completely converted to codeine following injection [2]. The highest median codeine concentration in the current study was observed with a PMI of 73–120 h after death (BNaF: 50 ng/mL, vitreous humor: 20 ng/mL).

4.4. Mode of Death

The use of blood-free morphine/total morphine ratios in the blood to identify the cause and mode of death has been reported [18,42]. However, this approach always involves certain issues. For example, morphine3-glucuronide and morphine-6-gluccronide are known to be unequal in terms of production and potency, and sample preparation using different hydrolysis procedures (acidic or enzymatic) seems to differ depending on the individual laboratory setting. The stability of morphine conjugates is affected by the phenomena of redistribution following death and enterohepatic recirculation. The total morphine content can be affected by the accumulation of morphine from previous injections. Therefore, free morphine is more important than total morphine for determining the blood concentrations of heroin-related fatalities [2,20,56].

Jones and Ahlner found no differences in the median blood morphine concentration between intoxication with polydrug and heroin-only [2]. Meissner et al. found that the median free morphine concentration was higher in polydrug intoxication than in heroin intoxication alone (232 ng/mL vs. 170 ng/mL, respectively) [57]. Al-Asmari reported that the median free morphine in heroin-only intoxication cases was marginally higher than that of multiple drug intoxication cases (152 vs. 108 ng/mL, respectively) [20].

This study is consistent with a previous investigation that found lower morphine concentrations when cocaine was co-administered [58]. The low free morphine concentration in blood in polydrug intoxication cases is consistent with a previous investigation that suggested that the possibility of overdose was potentially increased with the presence of other CNS drugs, even with low free morphine concentrations, due to the cumulative effects of these drugs, including heroin [59]. In contrast, in the presence of both cocaine and heroin, a higher free morphine concentration was obtained because both drugs are metabolized by carboxylesterases [58], which may inhibit the formation of morphine conjugates [19].

In this study, few case were positive for heroin and ethanol, where ethanol was attributed to antemortem ethanol ingestion. Moreover, the few cases may have been related to the low sample size of heroin users and the prohibition on ethanol intake by law in Saudi Arabia due to religious reasons [11,60]. In contrast, 28% and 13% of heroin cases showed co-ingestion of cannabinoids and amphetamine, respectively, which are more popular drugs in this region [25]; however, these drugs rarely contribute to death [61–63]. 6-MAM was detected in BNaF in most cases that tested positive for antemortem ethanol, which is consistent with the results of previous investigations [19].

Notably, Figure 2 shows the median concentration of morphine per year. In 2018, there were more cases but much lower concentrations than in 2014. The highest morphine concentration was observed in the current study despite having the fewest cases, and this can be interpreted as follows. In 2014, most cases involved mono-heroin intoxication, and almost 60% of cases were putrefied, which explains the high concentration of BNaF. In contrast, cases in 2018 comprised polydrug intoxication, including methamphetamine, cocaine, and tramadol, and only 20% of cases presented with slight putrefaction. In this project, a shift from mono-intoxication to intoxication from 2008, when this project was started, to a poly-drug intoxication trend at the end of this report in 2018, was observed.

In 2018, alprazolam was detected in 4 out of 15 cases; most of these cases involved polydrug intoxication, including methamphetamine, cocaine, and tramadol. In Saudi Arabia, alprazolam is a controlled drug, although the alprazolam supply has increased in illegal markets, which explains this increase. A similar trend has been observed with methamphetamine-related postmortem deaths in Jeddah, Saudi Arabia, in the same period [64]. Abuse of alprazolam and heroin has been previously reported, which reflects a high number of prescriptions or supplies from the illegal market [65]. In addition, few deaths related to alprazolam have been reported in the literature; however, intoxication cases with alprazolam and other drugs, especially cocaine, have been reported [66].

4.5. Time Span between Heroin Intake and Death

Consistent with previous reports, deaths following heroin intake can be divided into three types: rapid and delayed deaths, and undetermined survival times [2,3,51]. Rapid deaths can be identified by the detection of 6-MAM in blood samples, fresh needle marks, and the presence of syringes attached to the deceased body or nearby [3,42,59]. In addition, valuable information on the last moment before death can be obtained from family, friends, or witnesses [13]. Negative blood samples for 6-MAM may indicate a longer time between death and heroin administration (delayed death), which is supported by the detection of 6-MAM in other specimens, such as vitreous humor, urine, and bile [20,67]. Rapid deaths were expected to occur within <3 h after administration based on the detectable 6-MAM in blood, while delayed deaths occurred >3 h after administration based on the absence of 6-MAM in blood but presence in other specimens [3,51,68,69].

Goldberger et al. reported similar findings to the current study and showed that a higher median free morphine concentration occurred for rapid deaths (1420 ng/mL) compared to delayed deaths (250 ng/mL), while the median morphine for undetermined survival time after ingestion (610 ng/mL) was higher than that for delayed deaths [70]. Recently, Jakobsson et al. reported on 35 acute heroin-related deaths and found that the median free morphine concentration was 350 ng/mL for rapid deaths and 130 ng/mL for delayed deaths, respectively. The authors suggested that this discrepancy can be ascribed to a high heroin dose in rapid deaths [42]. This hypothesis is supported by the results from the current study and a previous investigation by Dark et al., who found that the median free morphine in rapid heroin death cases (260 ng/mL) was double that of delayed death cases (120 ng/mL) [58]. In addition, in some undetermined cases, the bodies were discovered many days after death, which increased the time between death and analysis. Such extended time periods were sufficient to convert 6-MAM and morphine conjugates to free morphine, which led to increased morphine concentrations in the blood. In contrast, in cases of delayed death, a considerable amount of morphine was eliminated before death, which resulted in low morphine concentrations [3].

The concentration of morphine in the vitreous humor is often lower than that in the blood. However, this concentration was found to be dependent on the survival time following heroin administration.

The use of the bile free morphine concentration to distinguish between rapid and delayed deaths has received little attention, and in most cases, the total morphine content has been reported. The total morphine concentration is significantly higher with delayed deaths, which indicates that the deceased is heroin-dependent and has received high doses of heroin [70]. The same observation was obtained in the current study, in which the bile free morphine concentration was higher in delayed death cases (2800 ng/mL) than in rapid (2200 ng/mL) and undetermined cases (1400 ng/mL). A similar finding has been reported regarding the role of urinalysis in cases of heroin-related deaths, with negative morphine or low concentrations used as an indicator of recent or naïve heroin use [71].

4.6. Manner of Death

In general, heroin-related deaths are most likely to occur due to accidental overdoses, although suicidal or homicidal modes of death have also been reported in the literature [13,69]. Abiragi et al. stated that identifying the mode of death in these cases is complicated if a relevant history of drug addiction and information on the last moment before death obtained from family or friends are not available at autopsy and in related toxicology reports [13]. One common finding was the lack of available information for individuals who were found dead without witnesses to the last moments before death. Gerostamoulos et al. [38] studied 434 heroin-related deaths in Victoria and found that 67% of these cases were found to be deceased, and 59% of the cases died alone. In that report, ambulances were called for 72% of the heroin-related deaths. Thaulow et al. studied 51 heroin-related deaths, and 64% of cases were found dead alone [3].

Depression is an indicator associated with heroin abuse, and it has led to an increase in violence-related deaths among heroin users [41,72]. Darke and Ross reported that the suicidal manner of heroin-related deaths ranges from 3% to −35% and suggested that heroin users are more prone to die by suicide at a rate 14-times higher than that of non-heroin users [72].

Opioids, such as heroin, are sedative drugs that are rarely associated with violence [72–74]. In cases where violence was attributed to heroin, it was considered indirect and not related to the effect of heroin ingestion; for example, it can arise from actions performed to obtain money for purchasing drugs [74]. A direct effect of heroin on homicide can be expected in the case of injecting or spiking heroin to sedate a victim because the dose may be higher than the victim can tolerate, or the user may be naive [74–76]. In addition, homicide deaths can occur between drug dealers, and violence also occurs between dealers and users [13,35,74]. Suicide-associated heroin deaths are underreported because it is difficult to differentiate between suicidal and accidental deaths based on the lack of necessary information from family and friends who may have witnessed the last moments of the deceased's life [13,72].

The median morphine concentration reported in this study was considered higher in cases of suicide-related deaths compared to those of accidental intoxication, which is consistent with the study by Darke et al. [41]. In most suicide cases, the method was a heroin overdose; deaths occurred in closed areas (home or prison); the deceased were male; and unemployment was a factor, which is consistent with prior investigations [72]. Moreover, the long history of heroin abuse reported in these cases may have increased the risk of depression, which led to suicidal thoughts. The highest morphine concentration reported in this study was for the suicide cases, which was consistent with the high blood morphine concentration (>1000 ng/mL) reported in a suicide case [41]. In another study that reported on two suicides by heroin injection, the blood morphine concentration was 630–640 ng/mL [77].

Heroin overdose as a means of homicide has been reported, and the percentages of heroin-related homicide have varied between studies. For example, in a study by Denninng et al., almost 20% of cases were reported to be homicides by drug overdose [78]. In other reports, ≥50% of homicide cases were due to the use of heroin as a means of intoxication [72,79–81]. In the current report, homicides were more frequent among younger users (median age: 22), while suicides were more frequent in older users (median age: 48), which is consistent with a previous report by Lee et al. [35]. Homicides cases frequently involved multiple drugs, and in the current study, all homicides cases were positive for cannabis, cocaine, tramadol, and alprazolam which is consistent with the findings of Lee et al. [35]. In contrast, suicide-related heroin cases mostly involve heroin alone. The most common cause of death is old age, which frequently involves other diseases due to prolonged heroin use, such as HIV and hepatitis, bronchopneumonia/acute pneumonia, cardiac problems, and a history of mental health problems [82,83]. Owing to the above-mentioned lack of drug abuse history and dying in deserted areas, which leads to putrefaction, an undetermined manner of death was recorded in 11% of the current cases. The manner of death in these cases was unknown due to a lack of information, and recent injection markers could not be found. Moreover, identifying the last injection site was difficult because most heroin addicts inject many times a day and most of the bodies were heavily decomposed. 6-MAM was only detected in blood samples from two of these cases.

4.7. Route of Administration

Our findings were consistent with the study by Thiblin et al. (median BNaF for injection = 230 ng/mL, non-injection = 100 ng/mL, and unknown routes of administration = 180 ng/mL) [84]. A higher median morphine concentration is often associated with heroin injection compared to non-injection routes. Consistent with the current investigation, Hadidi et al. concluded that the main route of heroin administration in Jorden was injection [36]. Crandall et al. [85] observed recent needle puncture marks in 77% of opioid overdose deaths, whereas drugs were found nearby in 51% of deaths. Darke and Duflou [58] reported that 44% of their cases died immediately, and needles or tourniquets were still attached to the bodies. In that study, 13% of the patients were transferred to the hospital. Thaulow et al. studied 51 heroin-related deaths, and syringes were discovered nearby the bodies in 16 out of 51 cases, with nine and seven classified as rapid and delayed deaths, respectively [3]. In a study from Thailand, needle puncture marks were observed in only 35% of deceased patients [86].

In the current study, no differences were observed in the median vitreous humor concentration among the three routes of administration. The most useful information obtained by measuring vitreous humor is the source of opiates administered when 6-MAM is detected in this matrix [4]. In contrast, Thaulow et al. [3] stated that the interpretation of the vitreous humor concentration of morphine can be complicated by many factors that make its use in postmortem investigations less suitable. One of the most obvious is the accumulation of morphine from a previous injection, especially for chronic users. In addition, it seems that the transport of morphine from the blood to the vitreous humor is slower, and a lag in distribution between these two matrices was reported [51]. Therefore, the use of morphine/codeine ratios to assess the source of opiates administered is not recommended. In the same report, using vitreous humor results, two cases were classified as codeine use if no 6-MAM was detected in the vitreous humor [3]. This is also complicated because the use of prescribed opiates and heroin together can increase this ratio and lead to misleading results. Therefore, no differences between different routes of administration can be expected due to the aforementioned factors. Darke and Ross reported a comparison between injection and non-injection in fetal heroin overdose cases. They found that a lack of differences between these two routes of administration and deaths due to heroin is not restricted to the injection of heroin and non-injection routes, along with the same heroin-overdose threat observed [87].

In a study by Fugelstad et al. [39], patients tested positive for HIV and hepatitis in 7.3% and 88% of cases, respectively. In a study from Victoria, 61% of the total cases tested positive for hepatitis, and only two cases were positive for HIV [38]. In another study, 50% of heroin-related deaths tested positive for hepatitis, and HIV was detected in 2% of the total cases [88].

It has been widely reported that heroin addiction is one of the main causes of HIV, and therefore, we believe that it is important to discuss the number of individuals who died from HIV. As the discussion here pertains to an epidemiological investigation in certain parts of the world for the first time, this piece of information is important. However, one of the limitations of this study is that the infectious disease history was not detailed in all cases. HIV and hepatitis were reported in fewer than 1% and 3% of total cases, respectively, which may indicate that sharing needles is not a common practice or that HIV deaths related to heroin addiction are under-reported in Saudi Arabia, considering that deaths due to infectious diseases are not usually subjected to postmortem analysis.

4.8. Location of Deaths and Putrefaction

The location where the bodies were found following a drug overdose is an important factor when interpreting the cause and manner of death. The impacts of ecological conditions, such as temperature and humidity, and location, such as indoor and outdoor places, on the analytes of interest in the postmortem samples were investigated. Few studies have discussed the location of heroin-related deaths. Fugelstad et al. [39] found that one-third of their cases occurred in private homes, almost 60% died alone with no witnesses, and only 9% were witnessed by others. In addition, Gerostamoulos et al. reported 434 heroin-related deaths in Victoria and showed that 60% occurred in the home [38]. In a study from Thailand, 40% and 24% of heroin-related deaths occurred in homes and hotels, respectively [86]. The risk of overdose increases when heroin is administered in public locations because the heroin users may inject the drug rapidly to avoid being noticed [88].

In previous studies, although putrefaction was reported, limited information regarding heroin-related metabolites was available. In the study by Crandall et al., putrefaction was observed in 12% of heroin-related deaths [85]. Crump et al. found that putrefaction degradation products did not interfere with morphine and codeine analyses [89]. Soravisut et al. concluded that morphine was detected in 50% of decomposed bodies in alternative specimens, such as liver tissues [86]. Reisinger et al. [90] compared oral cavity specimens with blood, urine, and bile specimens in cases of heroin-related fatalities. Some of these cases were partially or heavily decomposed (PMI 2–10 days). In their study, 6-MAM was found in the blood or urine of putrefied cases in 6 of 11 cases, which is consistent with the current investigation.

4.9. Seasonal Distribution

The impact of seasonal variation on heroin biomarkers and their metabolite analysis is believed to be a crucial factor underlying heroin-related deaths, especially in countries such as Saudi Arabia, where hot weather is more dominant. Kringsholm et al. [91] reported 205 heroin deaths and found that seasonal variations were not significant in most of the tested specimens. However, the weather in Denmark is cold [91] compared to that of Saudi Arabia. The detection of 6-MAM and 6-AC in bile seems to be seasonally dependent, despite the low sample size for bile, and the most frequent detections of these metabolites occurred in January and February. This can be attributed to stability issues for heroin biomarkers during the winter in Saudi Arabia. Soravisut et al. studied 142 opiate-related fatalities and found that the highest number of overdose deaths occurred in May [86].

4.10. Multiple Specimens

In forensic postmortem procedures, the ratio of morphine to codeine is of paramount importance in differentiating the source of opioid ingestion. A morphine-to-codeine ratio of less than one is considered an indicator of the intake of medicine containing codeine, while a morphine-to-codeine ratio of more than one is related to the use of heroin [3,51,92]. The interpretation of morphine/codeine ratios in the blood becomes difficult if morphine and heroin are administered. It is recommended to use these ratios in cases where no 6-MAM is detected; moreover, heroin intake can be confirmed if this ratio is higher than one and supported by information from the scene and autopsy findings [3,51]. Berg-Pedersen et al. studied the codeine/morphine ratio under different storage conditions and found that codeine and its glucuronide are more stable than morphine and its glucuronide in antemortem and postmortem cases [93]. Skopp et al. found that morphine conjugates were stable in the blood if they were subjected to proper storage at $-20\,°C$; however, increases in morphine were observed with heroin and codeine intoxication [94]. Morphine-3-glucuronide and morphine-6-glucuronide are cleavage products of morphine, and this cleavage occurs during sample storage, which increases the morphine concentration and affects the ratio between morphine and codeine [95,96]. In this study, the free morphine/codeine ratios were higher than 11, which agrees with previous investigations on heroin-related administration [20,97].

Many factors that affect the connections between heroin biomarkers and their metabolites must be taken into consideration, such as the history of abuse, concomitant use of other drugs, tolerance, route of administration, and PMI [3,33,44]. Mercurio et al. [98] studied 52 morphine-related deaths in which blood and bile were assessed in parallel and found that bile/blood morphine concentrations were poorly correlated ($r^2 = 0.01$, $p = 0.4$), which agrees with the current investigation. In that study, the median ratio of free morphine between the bile and blood was twenty-nine, which was lower than that in the current study. Duflou et al. reported the total morphine in blood and bile, and a strong correlation for the total morphine between blood and bile was obtained when using their data, with Rs = 0.712 and a p-value of 3×10^{-5}, and the median ratio of free morphine between bile and blood was 37 [96]. The morphine concentration in bile and urine was utilized to investigate whether the deceased had a history of heroin use, and in a previous study, heroin-related deaths were compared between two cities in the USA. In that study, blood morphine concentrations were similar, and both bile and urine provided information that users in San Francisco (n = 27 cases) were heroin-dependent while those in Connecticut (n = 15 cases) were naive or had stopped using heroin for some time before the last injection [54]. Negative or low concentrations of morphine in urine can be expected with rapid deaths related to heroin; for example, in two suicide-related heroin overdoses, the total morphine ranged from 100 to 500 ng/mL [77]. A low morphine concentration <1000 ng/mL is considered an indicator of a short survival time following heroin injection [71]. In addition, Jakobsson et al. compared heroin-related metabolites in urine with the findings of previous reports using free morphine and concluded that a higher concentration of urine free morphine is an indicator of a higher heroin dose [42].

The correlation of morphine in the blood with the vitreous humor has been widely studied. Scott and Oliver [52] found that this correlation was dependent on the rate of death and reported a good correlation ($r^2 = 0.697$) in all cases, whereas a strong correlation was obtained in 17 cases when the deaths were described as sudden ($r^2 = 0.885$). The same observation was reported by Rees et al. [51], who found a significant correlation for free morphine between the blood and vitreous humor, with Rs = 0.81 for rapid death and Rs = 0.71 for delayed death. In the current investigation, rapid death cases showed a better correlation (Rs = 0.650, $p = 8.0 \times 10^{-7}$) than delayed death cases (Rs = 0.450, $p = 0.1$).

5. Conclusions

To the best of our knowledge, this is the first epidemiological study evaluating heroin-related deaths in Jeddah, Saudi Arabia. Although the weather in Saudi Arabia is extremely hot most of the year, 6-MAM hydrolysis to morphine is favored. The detection of heroin biomarkers (6-MAM and 6-AC) is facilitated by short PMI periods in the majority of cases; moreover, the addition of sodium fluoride as a preservative prevents 6-MAM from being degraded to morphine in most cases. In addition, the availability of urine, vitreous humor, and bile samples provides valuable information on which opioids have been administered based on the detection of heroin biomarkers. The latter is important if no blood samples are available, if blood samples are negative for heroin biomarkers, and in cases of partially and heavily decomposed bodies. The incidence of heroin deaths in Jeddah remained stable during the study period. Most individual deaths likely occurred within groups, but the body was left behind or moved owing to fear among users to call an ambulance. Although only 24% of the deceased had medical records, the findings indicated an improvement in health reporting regarding drug abuse in Saudi Arabia. It is highly recommended that heroin users be encouraged to contact ambulances and trained in resuscitation. This study concluded that most patients were unemployed (up to 53%), had started taking heroin in their teens, and had been admitted several times to the addiction center. Therefore, the loss of tolerance following detoxification might have been the primary cause of many heroin-related deaths.

Supplementary Materials: The following supporting information can be downloaded at: https://www.mdpi.com/article/10.3390/toxics11030248/s1, Table S1: Summary of method validation parameters for the analysis of heroin biomarkers and their metabolites in blood, urine, vitreous humor, and bile; Table S2: Year distribution of 6-monoacetylmorphine, 6-acetylcodeine, morphine, and codeine in the 97 heroin-related deaths reported in Jeddah, Saudi Arabia, between 2008–2018; Table S3: Age distribution in the 97 heroin-related deaths examined in Jeddah, Saudi Arabia, between 2008–2018; Table S4: Concentrations of heroin biomarkers, morphine, and codeine in the 97 heroin related deaths in the current study according to post-mortem interval time group; Table S5: Comparison between heroin related metabolites concentrations in different bodily fluids according to the presence of injection marks at autopsy, presence of heroin materials in the scene and whether the last moment before death had been witnessed or they died alone in 97 heroin-related deaths in the current study; Table S6: Seasonal variation on the concentrations of heroin biomarkers, morphine, and codeine in the 97 heroin-related deaths in the current study; Table S7: Correlation between the heroin biomarkers, morphine, and codeine concentrations in the 97 heroin-related deaths in the current study; Figure S1: Variation of morphine concentration group in the blood with sodium fluoride (ng/mL) in the 97 heroin-related fatality cases in relation to postmortem interval time; Figure S2: Comparison between the median 6-monoacetylmorphine (ng/mL) in (a) blood with sodium fluoride and (b) vitreous humor samples in heroin-related deaths in the current study in relation to postmortem interval time; Figure S3: Distribution of heroin-related deaths in Jeddah, Saudi Arabia, between 2008–2018 (by month).

Author Contributions: Conceptualization, A.I.A.-A.; methodology, A.I.A.-A.; A.E.A.-Z., H.A., and T.A.Z.; software, A.E.A.-Z., T.A.Z., and H.A.; validation, A.I.A.-A., A.E.A.-Z., and H.A.; formal analysis, T.A.Z.; investigation, A.I.A.-A.; resources, A.E.A.-Z. and H.A.; data curation, A.I.A.-A., A.E.A.-Z., and H.A.; writing—original draft preparation, A.I.A.-A.; writing—review and editing, T.A.Z.; visualization, A.I.A.-A. and T.A.Z.; supervision, A.I.A.-A. and T.A.Z.; project administration, A.I.A.-A.; All authors have read and agreed to the published version of the manuscript.

Funding: This research received no external funding.

Institutional Review Board Statement: The study was conducted in accordance with the Declaration of Helsinki and approved by the Ethics Committee of Jeddah health Affair, Ministry of Health in Saudi Arabia, research code: 00188 (6 June 2014).

Informed Consent Statement: Not applicable.

Data Availability Statement: The data underlying this article will be shared on reasonable request with the corresponding author.

Acknowledgments: The authors would like to thank all the staff at the Forensic Toxicology Department-Jeddah Poison Control and Forensic Medical Chemistry Center for supporting this work.

Conflicts of Interest: The authors have no conflict of interest to declare.

References

1. United Nation Office on Drugs and Crime. *World Drug Report 2022*; United Nations Publication: Vienna, Austria, 2022; Available online: https://www.unodc.org/unodc/en/data-and-analysis/world-drug-report-2022.html (accessed on 20 January 2023).
2. Jones, A.W.; Holmgren, A.; Ahlner, J. Concentrations of Free-Morphine in Peripheral Blood after Recent Use of Heroin in Overdose Deaths and in Apprehended Drivers. *Forensic Sci. Int.* **2012**, *215*, 18–24. [CrossRef]
3. Thaulow, C.H.; Øiestad, Å.M.L.; Rogde, S.; Andersen, J.M.; Høiseth, G.; Handal, M.; Mørland, J.; Vindenes, V. Can Measurements of Heroin Metabolites in Post-Mortem Matrices Other than Peripheral Blood Indicate If Death Was Rapid or Delayed? *Forensic Sci. Int.* **2018**, *290*, 121–128. [CrossRef]
4. Maskell, P.D.; Wilson, N.E.; Seetohul, L.N.; Crichton, M.L.; Beer, L.J.; Drummond, G.; de Paoli, G. Postmortem Tissue Distribution of Morphine and Its Metabolites in a Series of Heroin-Related Deaths. *Drug Test. Anal.* **2019**, *11*, 292–304. [CrossRef] [PubMed]
5. European Monitoring Center for Drugs and Drug Addiction, Drug-Related Deaths and Mortality Rates in Europe. 2019. Available online: https://www.emcdda.europa.eu/topics/drug-related-deaths_en (accessed on 20 January 2023).
6. Evans, A.; Krause, M.; Leach, S.; Levitas, M.; Nguyen, L.; Short, L.C. Analysis of Drug Residue in Needle-Exchange Syringes in Washington, D.C. *Forensic Sci. Int.* **2021**, *329*, 111083. [CrossRef] [PubMed]
7. Drug Enforcement Administration. 2020 National Drug Threat Assessment (NDTA). Available online: https://www.dea.gov/sites/default/files/2021-02/DIR-008-21%202020%20National%20Drug%20Threat%20Assessment_WEB.pdf (accessed on 20 February 2023).
8. Bassiony, M. Substance Use Disorders in Saudi Arabia: Review Article. *J. Subst. Use* **2013**, *18*, 450–466. [CrossRef]
9. Osman, A.A. Substance Abuse among Patients Attending a Psychiatric Hospital in Jeddah: A Descriptive Study. *Ann. Saudi Med.* **1992**, *12*, 289–293. [CrossRef]
10. Al-Matrouk, A.; Al-Hasan, M.; Naqi, H.; Al-Abkal, N.; Mohammed, H.; Haider, M.; Al-Shammeri, D.; Bojbarah, H. Snapshot of Narcotic Drugs and Psychoactive Substances in Kuwait: Analysis of Illicit Drugs Use in Kuwait from 2015 to 2018. *BMC Public Health* **2021**, *21*, 671. [CrossRef]
11. Al-Asmari, A.I.; Al-Amoudi, D.H. The Role of Ethanol in Fatalities in Jeddah, Saudi Arabia. *Forensic Sci. Int.* **2020**, *316*, 110464. [CrossRef]
12. Al-Asmari, A.I. Applications of LC-MS/MS in Forensic Toxicology for the Analysis of Drugs and Their Metabolites. Ph.D. Dissertation, University of Glasgow, Glasgow, UK, 2009.
13. Abiragi, M.; Bauler, L.D.; Brown, T. Importance and Approach to Manner of Death Opinions in Opioid-Related Deaths. *J. Forensic Sci.* **2020**, *65*, 1009–1011. [CrossRef]
14. Elfawal, M.A. Trends in Fatal Substance Overdose in Eastern Saudi Arabia. *J. Clin. Forensic Med.* **1999**, *6*, 30–34. [CrossRef]
15. Maas, A.; Madea, B.; Hess, C. Confirmation of Recent Heroin Abuse: Accepting the Challenge. *Drug Test. Anal.* **2018**, *10*, 54–71. [CrossRef]
16. Pragst, F.; Spiegel, K.; Leuschner, U.; Hager, A. Detection of 6-Acetylmorphine in Vitreous Humor and Cerebrospinal Fluid-Comparison with Urinary Analysis for Proving Heroin Administration in Opiate Fatalities. *J. Anal. Toxicol.* **1999**, *23*, 168–172. [CrossRef] [PubMed]
17. Brenneisen, R.; Hasler, F.; Würsch, D. Acetylcodeine as a Urinary Marker to Differentiate the Use of Street Heroin and Pharmaceutical Heroin. *J. Anal. Toxicol.* **2002**, *26*, 561–566. [CrossRef]
18. Staub, C.; Jeanmonod, R.; Frye, O. Morphine in Postmortem Blood: Its Importance for the Diagnosis of Deaths Associated with Opiate Addiction. *Int. J. Leg. Med.* **1990**, *104*, 39–42. [CrossRef] [PubMed]
19. Al-Asmari, A.I.; Anderson, R.A. Method for Quantification of Opioids and Their Metabolites in Autopsy Blood by Liquid Chromatography-Tandem Mass Spectrometry. *J. Anal. Toxicol.* **2007**, *31*, 394–408. [CrossRef]
20. Al-Asmari, A.I. Postmortem Fluid Concentrations of Heroin Biomarkers and Their Metabolites. *J. Forensic Sci.* **2020**, *65*, 570–579. [CrossRef]
21. Al-Asmari, A.I.; Alharbi, H.; Zughaibi, T.A. Post-Mortem Analysis of Heroin Biomarkers, Morphine and Codeine in Stomach Wall Tissue in Heroin-Related Deaths. *Toxics* **2022**, *10*, 473. [CrossRef]
22. *ANSI/ASB Standard 036*; American Academy of Forensic Sciences Standards Board 2019. Method Validation in Forensic Toxicology: Colorado Springs, CO, USA, 2019.
23. Bidny, S.; Gago, K.; Chung, P.; Albertyn, D.; Pasin, D. Simultaneous Screening and Quantification of Basic, Neutral and Acidic Drugs in Blood Using UPLC-QTOF-MS. *J. Anal. Toxicol.* **2017**, *41*, 181–195. [CrossRef] [PubMed]
24. Di Rago, M.; Saar, E.; Rodda, L.N.; Turfus, S.; Kotsos, A.; Gerostamoulos, D.; Drummer, O.H. Fast Targeted Analysis of 132 Acidic and Neutral Drugs and Poisons in Whole Blood Using LC-MS/MS. *Forensic Sci. Int.* **2014**, *243*, 35–43. [CrossRef]

25. Al-Asmari, A.I. Method for the Identification and Quantification of Sixty Drugs and Their Metabolites in Postmortem Whole Blood Using Liquid Chromatography Tandem Mass Spectrometry. *Forensic Sci. Int.* **2020**, *309*, 110193. [CrossRef]
26. Maurer, H.H. Chapter 12 Forensic Screening with GC-MS. *Handb. Anal. Sep.* **2008**, *6*, 425–445. [CrossRef]
27. Wylie, F.M.; Torrance, H.; Seymour, A.; Buttress, S.; Oliver, J.S. Drugs in Oral Fluid: Part II. Investigation of Drugs in Drivers. *Forensic Sci. Int.* **2005**, *150*, 199–204. [CrossRef] [PubMed]
28. Matuszewski, B.K.; Constanzer, M.L.; Chavez-Eng, C.M. Strategies for the Assessment of Matrix Effect in Quantitative Bioanalytical Methods Based on HPLC-MS/MS. *Anal. Chem.* **2003**, *75*, 3019–3030. [CrossRef] [PubMed]
29. Peters, F.T.; Drummer, O.H.; Musshoff, F. Validation of New Methods. *Forensic Sci. Int.* **2007**, *165*, 216–224. [CrossRef] [PubMed]
30. Kintz, P.; Jamey, C.; Cirimele, V.; Brenneisen, R.; Ludes, B. Evaluation of Acetylcodeine as a Specific Marker of Illicit Heroin in Human Hair. *J. Anal. Toxicol.* **1998**, *22*, 425–429. [CrossRef] [PubMed]
31. Staub, C.; Marset, M.; Mino, A.; Mangin, P. Detection of Acetylcodeine in Urine as an Indicator of Illicit Heroin Use: Method Validation and Results of a Pilot Study. *Clin. Chem.* **2001**, *47*, 301–307. [CrossRef]
32. O'Neal, C.L.; Poklis, A. Postmortem Production of Ethanol and Factors That Influence Interpretation: A Critical Review. *Am. J. Forensic Med. Pathol.* **1996**, *17*, 8–20. [CrossRef]
33. Al-Asmari, A.I.; Altowairgi, M.M.; Al-Amoudi, D.H. Effects of Postmortem Interval, Putrefaction, Diabetes, and Location of Death on the Analysis of Ethyl Glucuronide and Ethyl Sulfate as Ethanol Biomarkers of Antemortem Alcohol Consumption. *Forensic Sci. Int.* **2022**, *335*, 111280. [CrossRef]
34. Steentoft, A.; Worm, K.; Christensen, H. Morphine Concentrations in Autopsy Material from Fatal Cases after Intake of Morphine and/or Heroin. *J. Forensic Sci. Soc.* **1988**, *28*, 87–94. [CrossRef]
35. Lee, D.; Delcher, C.; Maldonado-Molina, M.M.; Thogmartin, J.R.; Goldberger, B.A. Manners of Death in Drug-Related Fatalities in Florida. *J. Forensic Sci.* **2016**, *61*, 735–742. [CrossRef]
36. Hadidi, M.S.; Ibrahim, M.I.; Abdallat, I.M.; Hadidi, K.A. Current Trends in Drug Abuse Associated Fatalities-Jordan, 2000–2004. *Forensic Sci. Int.* **2009**, *186*, 44–47. [CrossRef] [PubMed]
37. Taghaddosinejad, F.; Arefi, M.; Fayaz, A.F.; Tanhaeivash, R. Determination of Substance Overdose in Two Iranian Centers: Comparison between Opioids and Non-Opioids. *J. Forensic Leg. Med.* **2013**, *20*, 155–157. [CrossRef] [PubMed]
38. Gerostamoulos, J.; Staikos, V.; Drummer, O.H. Heroin-Related Deaths in Victoria: A Review of Cases for 1997 and 1998. *Drug Alcohol Depend.* **2001**, *61*, 123–127. [CrossRef] [PubMed]
39. Fugelstad, A.; Ahlner, J.; Brandt, L.; Ceder, G.; Eksborg, S.; Rajs, J.; Beck, O. Use of Morphine and 6-Monoacetylmorphine in Blood for the Evaluation of Possible Risk Factors for Sudden Death in 192 Heroin Users. *Addiction* **2003**, *98*, 463–470. [CrossRef] [PubMed]
40. Burt, M.J.; Kloss, J.; Apple, F.S. Postmortem Blood Free and Total Morphine Concentrations in Medical Examiner Cases. *J. Forensic Sci.* **2001**, *46*, 1138–1142. [CrossRef] [PubMed]
41. Darke, S.; Duflou, J.; Torok, M. Comparative Toxicology of Intentional and Accidental Heroin Overdose. *J. Forensic Sci.* **2010**, *55*, 1015–1018. [CrossRef]
42. Jakobsson, G.; Truver, M.T.; Wrobel, S.A.; Gréen, H.; Kronstrand, R. Heroin-Related Compounds and Metabolic Ratios in Postmortem Samples Using LC-MS-MS. *J. Anal. Toxicol.* **2021**, *45*, 215–225. [CrossRef]
43. Frost, J.; Løkken, T.N.; Helland, A.; Nordrum, I.S.; Slørdal, L. Post-Mortem Levels and Tissue Distribution of Codeine, Codeine-6-Glucuronide, Norcodeine, Morphine and Morphine Glucuronides in a Series of Codeine-Related Deaths. *Forensic Sci. Int.* **2016**, *262*, 128–137. [CrossRef]
44. Skopp, G. Postmortem Toxicology. *Forensic Sci. Med. Pathol.* **2010**, *6*, 314–325. [CrossRef]
45. Gerostamoulos, J.; Drummer, O.H. Postmortem Redistribution of Morphine and Its Metabolites. *J. Forensic Sci.* **2000**, *45*, 843–845. [CrossRef]
46. Logan, B.K.; Smirnow, D. Postmortem Distribution and Redistribution of Morphine in Man. *J. Forensic Sci.* **1996**, *41*, 37–46. [CrossRef]
47. Sawyer, W.R.; Forney, R.B. Postmortem Disposition of Morphine in Rats. *Forensic Sci. Int.* **1988**, *38*, 259–273. [CrossRef] [PubMed]
48. Degouffe, M.; Drost, M. A Comparison of Drug Concentrations in Postmortem Cardiac and Peripheral Blood in 320 Cases. *J. Can. Soc. Forensic Sci.* **1995**, *28*, 113–121. [CrossRef]
49. Maskell, P.D.; Albeishy, M.; de Paoli, G.; Wilson, N.E.; Seetohul, L.N. Postmortem Redistribution of the Heroin Metabolites Morphine and Morphine-3-Glucuronide in Rabbits over 24 h. *Int. J. Leg. Med.* **2016**, *130*, 519–531. [CrossRef] [PubMed]
50. Romberg, R.W.; Lee, L. Comparison of the Hydrolysis Rates of Morphine-3-Glucuronide and Morphine-6-Glucuronide with Acid and β-Glucuronidase. *J. Anal. Toxicol.* **1995**, *19*, 157–162. [CrossRef]
51. Rees, K.A.; Pounder, D.J.; Osselton, M.D. Distribution of Opiates in Femoral Blood and Vitreous Humour in Heroin/Morphine-Related Deaths. *Forensic Sci. Int.* **2013**, *226*, 152–159. [CrossRef]
52. Scott, K.S.; John, G.; Oliver, S.; Frsc, C. Vitreous Humor as an Alternative Sample to Blood for the Supercritical Fluid Extraction of Morphine and 6-Monoacetylmorphine. *Med. Sci. Law* **1999**, *39*, 77–81. [CrossRef]
53. Moffat, A.C.; Osselton, M.D.; Widdop, B. Diamorphine. In *Clarke's Analysis of Drugs and Poisons in Pharmaceuticals, Body Fluids and Postmortem Material*, 4th ed.; Pharmaceutical Press: London, UK, 2011; pp. 1225–1227.
54. Baselt, R.C.; Cravey, R.H. Heroin. In *Disposition of Toxic Drugs and Chemicals in Man*, 11th ed.; Baselt, R.C., Ed.; Biomedical Publications: Foster City, CA, USA, 2020; pp. 1031–1036.

55. Nassibou, S.; Richeval, C.; Wiart, J.F.; Hakim, F.; Allorge, D.; Gaulier, J.M. In Heroin-Related Fatalities, Testing for 6-Acetylmorphine in Vitreous Humor Seems to Be of Higher Sensitivity than in Blood or Urine. *J. Anal. Toxicol.* **2020**, *44*, E9–E10. [CrossRef]
56. Jones, A.W.; Holmgren, A.; Ahlner, J. Heroin Poisoning Deaths with 6-Acetylmorphine in Blood: Demographics of the Victims, Previous Drug-Related Offences, Polydrug Use, and Free Morphine Concentrations in Femoral Blood. *Forensic Toxicol.* **2012**, *30*, 19–24. [CrossRef]
57. Meissner, C.; Recker, S.; Reiter, A.; Friedrich, H.J.; Oehmichen, M. Fatal versus Non-Fatal Heroin "Overdose": Blood Morphine Concentrations with Fatal Outcome in Comparison to Those of Intoxicated Drivers. *Forensic Sci. Int.* **2002**, *130*, 49–54. [CrossRef]
58. Polettini, A.; Poloni, V.; Groppi, A.; Stramesi, C.; Vignali, C.; Politi, L.; Montagna, M. The Role of Cocaine in Heroin-Related Deaths: Hypothesis on the Interaction between Heroin and Cocaine. *Forensic Sci. Int.* **2005**, *153*, 23–28. [CrossRef] [PubMed]
59. Darke, S.; Duflou, J. The Toxicology of Heroin-Related Death: Estimating Survival Times. *Addiction* **2016**, *111*, 1607–1613. [CrossRef] [PubMed]
60. The Saudi Food and Drug Authority Regulations and Regulations for General Provisions on Schedules Attached to the Anti-Drug and Psychotropic Substances System. *Um Alqura Newspaper*, 2019.
61. Logan, B.K.; Fligner, C.L.; Haddix, T. Cause and Manner of Death in Fatalities Involving Methamphetamine. *J. Forensic Sci.* **1998**, *43*, 28–34. [CrossRef] [PubMed]
62. Darke, S.; Duflou, J.; Lappin, J.; Kaye, S. Clinical and Autopsy Characteristics of Fatal Methamphetamine Toxicity in Australia. *J. Forensic Sci.* **2018**, *63*, 1466–1471. [CrossRef] [PubMed]
63. Al-Asmari, A.I.; Al-Solami, F.D.; Al-Zahrani, A.E.; Zughaibi, T.A. Post-Mortem Quantitation of Amphetamine in Cadaveric Fluids in Saudi Arabia. *Forensic Sci.* **2022**, *2*, 222–237. [CrossRef]
64. Al-Asmari, A.I. Methamphetamine-Related Postmortem Cases in Jeddah, Saudi Arabia. *Forensic Sci. Int.* **2021**, *321*, 110746. [CrossRef]
65. Rintoul, A.C.; Dobbin, M.D.H.; Nielsen, S.; Degenhardt, L.; Drummer, O.H. Recent Increase in Detection of Alprazolam in Victorian Heroin-Related Deaths. *Med. J. Aust.* **2013**, *198*, 206–209. [CrossRef]
66. Wolf, B.C.; Lavezzi, W.A.; Sullivan, L.M.; Middleberg, R.A.; Flannagan, L.M. Alprazolam-Related Deaths in Palm Beach County. *Am. J. Forensic Med. Pathol.* **2005**, *26*, 24–27. [CrossRef]
67. Thaulow, C.H.; Øiestad, Å.M.L.; Rogde, S.; Karinen, R.; Brochmann, G.W.; Andersen, J.M.; Høiseth, G.; Handal, M.; Mørland, J.; Arnestad, M.; et al. Metabolites of Heroin in Several Different Post-Mortem Matrices. *J. Anal. Toxicol.* **2018**, *42*, 311–320. [CrossRef]
68. Spiehler, V.; Brown, R. Unconjugated Morphine in Blood by Radioimmunoassay and Gas Chromatography/Mass Spectrometry. *J. Forensic Sci.* **1987**, *32*, 906–916. [CrossRef]
69. Garriott, J.C.; Sturner, W.Q. Morphine Concentrations and Survival Periods in Acute Heroin Fatalities. *N. Engl. J. Med.* **1973**, *289*, 1276–1278. [CrossRef] [PubMed]
70. Goldberger, B.A.; Cone, E.J.; Grant, T.M.; Levine, B.S.; Smialek, J.E. Disposition of Heroin and Its Metabolites in Heroin-Related Deaths. *J. Anal. Toxicol.* **1994**, *18*, 22–28. [CrossRef]
71. Singer, R. The Forensic Pharmacology of Drugs of Abuse. *Int. J. Toxicol.* **2002**, *21*, 436–437. [CrossRef]
72. Darke, S.; Ross, J. Suicide among Heroin Users: Rates, Risk Factors and Methods. *Addiction* **2002**, *97*, 1383–1394. [CrossRef] [PubMed]
73. Concool, B.; Smith, H.; Stimmel, B. Mortality Rates of Persons Entering Methadone Maintenance: A Seven-Year Study. *Am. J. Drug Alcohol Abus.* **1979**, *6*, 345–353. [CrossRef]
74. Darke, S. The Toxicology of Homicide Offenders and Victims: A Review. *Drug Alcohol Rev.* **2010**, *29*, 202–215. [CrossRef]
75. Paul, A.B.M.; Simms, L.; Mahesan, A.M. Intentional Heroin Administration Resulting in Homicide in a 10-Month Old Infant. *Forensic Sci. Int.* **2018**, *290*, e15–e18. [CrossRef]
76. Missliwetz, J.; Vycudilik, W. Homicide by Strangling or Dumping with Postmortem Injuries after Heroin Poisoning? *Am. J. Forensic Med. Pathol.* **1997**, *18*, 211–214. [CrossRef]
77. Reed, D.; Spiehler, V.R.; Cravey, R.H. Two Cases of Heroin-Related Suicide. *Forensic Sci.* **1977**, *9*, 49–52. [CrossRef]
78. Denning, D.G.; Conwell, Y.; King, D.; Cox, C. Method Choice, Intent, and Gender in Completed Suicide. *Suicide Life Threat. Behav.* **2000**, *30*, 282–288.
79. Marx, A.; Schick, M.T.; Minder, C.E. Drug-Related Mortality in Switzerland from 1987 to 1989 in Comparison to Other Countries. *Int. J. Addict.* **1994**, *29*, 837–860. [CrossRef] [PubMed]
80. Rossow, I. Suicide among Drug Addicts in Norway. *Addiction* **1994**, *89*, 1667–1673. [CrossRef] [PubMed]
81. Dukes, P.D.; Robinson, G.M.; Robinson, B.J. Mortality of Intravenous Drug Users: Attenders of the Wellington Drug Clinic, 1972–1989. *Drug Alcohol Rev.* **1992**, *11*, 197–201. [CrossRef] [PubMed]
82. Stam, N.C.; Gerastamoulos, D.; Pilgrim, J.L.; Smith, K.; Moran, L. Letter to the Editor Drug-Related Deaths-A Wider View Is Necessary. *Addiction* **2019**, *114*, 1504. [CrossRef]
83. Roxburgh, A.; Pilgrim, J.L.; Hall, W.D.; Burns, L.; Degenhardt, L. Accurate Identification of Opioid Overdose Deaths Using Coronial Data. *Forensic Sci. Int.* **2018**, *287*, 40–46. [CrossRef]
84. Thiblin, I.; Eksborg, S.; Petersson, A.; Fugelstad, A.; Rajs, J. Fatal Intoxication as a Consequence of Intranasal Administration (Snorting) or Pulmonary Inhalation (Smoking) of Heroin. *Forensic Sci. Int.* **2004**, *139*, 241–247. [CrossRef]

85. Crandall, C.S.; Kerrigan, S.; Aguero, R.L.; LaValley, J.; McKinney, P.E. The Influence of Collection Site and Methods on Postmortem Morphine Concentrations in a Porcine Model. *J. Anal. Toxicol.* **2006**, *30*, 651–658. [CrossRef] [PubMed]
86. Soravisut, N.; Rattanasalee, P.; Junkuy, A.; Thampitak, S.; Sribanditmongkol, P. Comparative Analysis of Pathological and Toxicological Features of Opiate Overdose and Non-Overdose Fatalities. *J. Med. Assoc. Thail. Chotmaihet Thangphaet* **2011**, *94*, 1540–1546.
87. Darke, S.; Ross, J. Fatal Heroin Overdoses Resulting from Non-Injecting Routes of Administration, NSW, Australia, 1992–1996. *Addiction* **2000**, *95*, 569–573. [CrossRef]
88. Warner-Smith, M.; Darke, S.; Lynskey, M.; Hall, W. Heroin Overdose: Causes and Consequences. *Addiction* **2001**, *96*, 1113–1125. [CrossRef]
89. Crump, K.L.; McIntyre, M.; Drummer, O.H. Simultaneous Determination of Morphine and Codeine in Blood and Bile Using Dual Ultraviolet and Fluorescence High-Performance Liquid Chromatography. *J. Anal. Toxicol.* **1994**, *18*, 208–212. [CrossRef]
90. Reisinger, A.J.; Miller, A.C.; Shaw, L.A.; Champion, J.L.; Neiswonger, M.A. Oral Cavity Fluid as an Investigative Approach for Qualitative and Quantitative Evaluations of Drugs in Postmortem Subjects. *J. Anal. Toxicol.* **2019**, *43*, 444–451. [CrossRef]
91. Kringsholm, B.; Voigt, J.; Dalgaard, J.B.; Simonsen, J. Deaths among Narcotic Addicts in Denmark in 1978 and 1979. *Forensic Sci. Int.* **1981**, *18*, 19–30. [CrossRef]
92. Jones, A.W.; Holmgren, A. Concentration Ratios of Free-Morphine to Free-Codeine in Femoral Blood in Heroin-Related Poisoning Deaths. *Leg. Med.* **2011**, *13*, 171–173. [CrossRef]
93. Berg-Pedersen, R.M.; Ripel, Å.; Karinen, R.; Vevelstad, M.; Bachs, L.; Vindenes, V. Codeine to Morphine Concentration Ratios in Samples from Living Subjects and Autopsy Cases after Incubation. *J. Anal. Toxicol.* **2014**, *38*, 99–105. [CrossRef]
94. Skopp, G.; Pötsch, L.; Klingmann, A.; Mattern, R. Stability of Morphine, Morphine-3-Glucuronide, and Morphine-6-Glucuronide in Fresh Blood and Plasma and Postmortem Blood Samples. *J. Anal. Toxicol.* **2001**, *25*, 2–7. [CrossRef]
95. Moriya, F.; Hashimoto, Y. Distribution of Free and Conjugated Morphine in Body Fluids and Tissues in a Fatal Heroin Overdose: Is Conjugated Morphine Stable in Postmortem Specimens? *J. Forensic Sci.* **1997**, *42*, 736–740. [CrossRef]
96. Duflou, J.; Darke, S.; Easson, J. Morphine Concentrations in Stomach Contents of Intravenous Opioid Overdose Deaths. *J. Forensic Sci.* **2009**, *54*, 1181–1184. [CrossRef]
97. Al-Asmari, A.I. Postmortem Liver and Kidney Tissue Concentrations of Heroin Biomarkers and Their Metabolites in Heroin-Related Fatalities. *J. Forensic Sci.* **2020**, *65*, 2087–2093. [CrossRef]
98. Mercurio, I.; Ceraso, G.; Melai, P.; Gili, A.; Troiano, G.; Agostinelli, F.; Lancia, M.; Bacci, M. Significance of Morphine Concentration in Bile, Liver, and Blood: Analysis of 52 Cases of Heroin Overdoses. *Am. J. Forensic Med. Pathol.* **2019**, *40*, 329–335. [CrossRef]

Disclaimer/Publisher's Note: The statements, opinions and data contained in all publications are solely those of the individual author(s) and contributor(s) and not of MDPI and/or the editor(s). MDPI and/or the editor(s) disclaim responsibility for any injury to people or property resulting from any ideas, methods, instructions or products referred to in the content.

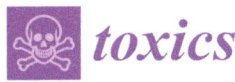

Article

Fatalities Involving Khat in Jazan, Saudi Arabia, 2018 to 2021

Ghassan Shaikhain [1], Mohammed Gaballah [2], Ahmad Alhazmi [2], Ibrahim Khardali [1], Ahmad Hakami [2], Magbool Oraiby [1], Sultan Alharbi [1], Mohammad Tobaigi [2], Mohammed Ghalibi [2], Mohsen Fageeh [1], Mohammed Albeishy [1] and Ibraheem Attafi [1,*]

[1] Forensic Toxicology Services, Forensic Medical Center, Ministry of Health, Jazan 45142, Saudi Arabia
[2] Forensic Medicine Services, Forensic Medical Center, Ministry of Health, Jazan 45142, Saudi Arabia
* Correspondence: iattafi@moh.gov.sa; Tel.: +966-1-591610440

Abstract: Interpreting fatalities involving khat is challenging due to a lack of data on cathinone and cathine reference concentrations in postmortem tissues. This study investigated the autopsy findings and toxicological results of fatalities involving khat in Saudi Arabia's Jazan region from 1 January 2018 to 31 December 2021. All confirmed cathine and cathinone results in postmortem blood, urine, brain, liver, kidney, and stomach samples were recorded and analyzed. Autopsy findings and the manner and cause of death of the deceased were assessed. Saudi Arabia's Forensic Medicine Center investigated 651 fatality cases over four years. Thirty postmortem samples were positive for khat's active constituents, cathinone and cathine. The percentage of fatalities involving khat was 3% in 2018 and 2019 and increased from 4% in 2020 to 9% in 2021, when compared with all fatal cases. They were all males ranging in age from 23 to 45. Firearm injuries (10 cases), hanging (7 cases), road traffic accident (2 cases), head injury (2 cases), stab wounds (2 cases), poisoning (2 cases), unknown (2 cases), ischemic heart disease (1 case), brain tumor (1 case), and choking (1 case) were responsible for the deaths. In total, 57% of the postmortem samples tested positive for khat only, while 43% tested positive for khat with other drugs. Amphetamine is the drug most frequently involved. The average cathinone and cathine concentrations were 85 and 486 ng/mL in the blood, 69 and 682 ng/mL in the brain, 64 and 635 ng/mL in the liver, and 43 and 758 ng/mL in the kidneys, respectively. The 10th–90th percentiles of blood concentrations of cathinone and cathine were 18–218 ng/mL and 222–843 ng/mL, respectively. These findings show that 90% of fatalities involving khat had cathinone concentrations greater than 18 ng/mL and cathine concentrations greater than 222 ng/mL. According to the cause of death, homicide was the most common fatality involving khat alone (77%). More research is required, especially toxicological and autopsy findings, to determine the involvement of khat in crimes and fatalities. This study may help forensic scientists and toxicologists investigate fatalities involving khat.

Keywords: forensic toxicology; khat; cathinone; cathine; postmortem

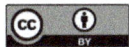

1. Introduction

Khat is the common name for the plant known by its scientific name as Catha edulis (Vahl) Forssk. ex Endl. Typically, its leaves are chewed to produce stimulant effects such as alertness, euphoria, and increased motor activity [1]. The two major active components of khat are cathine and cathinone. They are listed in the controlled substances act as psychotropic substances Schedules III and I, respectively, and the khat plant is listed as a controlled plant [2]. Despite the low concentrations of cathine and cathinone in khat leaves (which range from 0.1% to 0.2% and from 0.1% to 0.3%, respectively), long-term consumption of large amounts of khat leaves can cause toxicity [3,4]. In addition to those compounds, khat leaves also contain sterols, tannins, cathedulins (polyhydroxylated sesquiterpenes), triterpenes, and flavonoids [5].

The most potentially toxic effects of khat consumption are hyperthermia, insomnia, anorexia, constipation, urinary retention, hypertension, myocardial infarction, and arrhythmia [6–9]. Hepatitis was also reported in two khat users, which was resolved by discontinuing khat use, but relapse occurred when khat use was resumed in both cases [10]. There are also reported cases of cerebral hemorrhage, psychoactive disorders, and cancer [5,11]. Chewers of khat typically consume 50–200 g of fresh khat leaves per day [12]. This amount of khat leaves consumed daily induces psychological dependence and tolerance, leading to an increased daily consumption [13–15]. The metabolic cytochrome P450 enzymes 3A4, 2D6, 2C19, and 1A2 are affected by khat consumption [16,17]. Hence, the inhibitory effects of khat on metabolic enzymes may alter plasma concentrations, which may impact the efficacy and safety of drug therapy.

Both cathine and cathinone are basic compounds with pKa values of 9.37 and 7.55, respectively, and are susceptible to postmortem redistribution [18]. As a parent drug, cathine and cathinone are excreted in human urine. Furthermore, they each have a minor metabolite, pseudoephedrine and diethylpropion [19,20]. Cathinone was also rapidly converted to norephedrine and nor-pseudoephedrine [21]. Consequently, the aforementioned metabolites may indicate Khat consumption [22].

The toxicity of khat exposure has been demonstrated by previous studies, and the possibility of lethality cannot be ruled out. To rule out an overdose as the cause of death, toxicologists must evaluate and interpret the substance concentrations present in postmortem samples. Substance concentrations must be quantified, reported, and published to expand the limited published evidence on toxicological findings for fatalities involving khat. The autopsy findings and other circumstances surrounding death are also important indicators of substance-related deaths. The results of an autopsy finding will also be important for figuring out what concentrations of cathine and cathinone are dangerous and which are fatal. Studying the prevalence of fatalities involving khat is also important for prevention, treatment, and education. The purpose of this study were (a) to analyze fatalities involving khat in Jazan, Saudi Arabia, and (b) to explore the disposition of cathine and cathinone in postmortem tissues.

2. Materials and Methods

2.1. Study Design and Data Collection

All fatal forensic cases received at the Poison Control and Medical Forensic Chemistry Center in Jazan, Saudi Arabia, from the 1st of January 2018 to the 31st of December 2021 were retrospectively evaluated. The data were collected from the OTARR electronic system using the data collection form. All acquired data regarding the toxicological study results and accident summary, including the manner of death in the forensic cases involving khat, were analyzed. These data included forensic cases that are confirmed as positive for the presence of cathine and cathinone and excluded the forensic cases that are negative for the presence of cathine and cathinone.

All information regarding the autopsy finding, manner, and causes of death in fatalities involving khat within the period of study was revised, defined, and recorded by the medical forensic examiner experts at the Jazan Forensic Medicine Center. The autopsy finding data in the autopsied cases were clearly defined and tabulated. The manner of death was classified as follows: suicidal, homicidal, accidental, and undetermined. The identification of hazards for cathine and cathinone, as well as forensic cases involving their exposure, have been evaluated.

2.2. Toxicological Analysis

Drugs of abuse including amphetamines, cocaine, cannabinoids, opiates, barbiturates, and benzodiazepines in all autopsied samples are primarily screened via immunoassay analysis using the RANDOX system (Evidence Plus; Randox Laboratories, Crumlin, UK). Volatiles including methanol, ethanol, isopropanol, and acetone are routinely analyzed using headspace-gas chromatography. Using liquid chromatography–mass spectrometry, the immunoassay positive results for amphetamine-type stimulants (including amphetamine, methamphetamine, cathine, and cathinone) were confirmed and quantified, while gas chromatography–mass spectrometry was used to exclude other drugs.

Cathine and cathinone concentrations were identified and quantified via the liquid chromatography–ion trap mass spectrometry (LCQ Fleet Ion Trap LC/MS) method (Thermo Fisher Scientific, Waltham, MA, USA). For sample preparation, one gram of each organ tissue was homogenized in one milliliter of deionized water and then centrifuged for 15 min at 3000× g using a Heraeus Labofuge 400 centrifuge (Thermo Fisher Scientific, Waltham, MA, USA). The supernatant was then mixed with 1 mL of phosphate buffer pH 6 and vortexed for solid phase extraction (SPE) using DAU extraction columns (UCT, Bristol, PA, USA). Prior to the extraction procedure, one milliliter of each sample's homogenate was spiked with 20 μL of a prepared stock solution of 3,4-methylenedioxymethamphetamine (MDMA) at a concentration of 50 μg/mL as an internal standard. SPE columns were preconditioned with 3 mL methanol and 3 mL deionized water and equilibrated with 1 mL phosphate buffer at pH 6. Upon sample load completion, SPE columns were washed with 3 mL of deionized water, 1 mL of 0.1 M acetic acid, and 3 mL of methanol and dried for 10 min under a nitrogen stream. Next, cathine, cathinone, and MDMA were eluted into 12 mL glass tubes with 3 mL of a mixture of dichloromethane, isopropanol, and ammonium hydroxide (78:20:2, $v:v:v$). Then, one drop of 0.1 M hydrochloric acid (HCl) was added into each tube, and all elutions were evaporated to dryness under nitrogen stream. Finally, all samples were reconstituted with 100 μL of the aqueous proportion of the mobile phase (10 mM ammonium formate with 0.11% formic acid) for LCQ Fleet Ion Trap LC/MS analysis.

Calibration samples were prepared by spiking 1 mL of blank tissue homogenates with cathine, cathinone, and MDMA (Lipomed, Arlesheim, Switzerland). Six calibration points were prepared at concentrations of 50, 100, 250, 500, 1000, 2000, 3000, 4000, and 6000 ng/mL of cathine and cathinone and 1000 ng/mL MDMA as the internal standard. Postmortem samples were diluted prior to extraction and reanalyzed when concentrations exceeded the upper limits of quantification. Three quality control samples were prepared by spiking 1 mL of the blank homogenate tissues with cathine and cathinone at the concentrations of 100, 250, and 500 ng/mL and the concentration of 1000 ng/mL of MDMA as an internal standard.

An LCQ Fleet Ion Trap LC/MS system (Thermo Fisher Scientific, Waltham, MA, USA), employing an LCQ fleet mass analyzer coupled with a Surveyor Auto-Sampler and a Surveyor Quaternary Pump and managed by X-Caliber Software (Themo Scientific, USA), was used. Briefly, 10 μL of each sample was injected by an autosampler. The chromatographic separation of cathine, cathinone, and MDMA was achieved with a HPLC column (Hypersil GOLD, 5 μm, 150 × 4.6 mm, Thermo Fisher Scientific, Waltham, MA, USA), using mobile phase A (ammonium formate (10 Mm; 0.639 mg ammonium formate in 1 L HPLC water) and mobile phase B (formic acid in acetonitrile (0.1%; 1 mL formic acid in 999 mL acetonitrile). Gradient elution was performed as follows: 0–1 min, 100% A; and 1–7.5 min, 80% A; 7.5–8.5 min, 50% A, 8.5–9.5 min, 0% A; 9.5–10.5 min, 50% A; and 10.5–11.5 min 100% A. Flow rate was 300 μL/min, and the injection volume was 5 μL. The electrospray ion source (ESI), as an optimized tuning profile of ATS, runs in positive ionization mode with 5 kV spraying voltage, 275 °C capillary temperature, and sheath gas value 30. The mass analyzer runs in the scan mode, scanning at m/z 152 for cathine, m/z 150 for cathinone, and m/z 194 for MDMA. Cathine, cathinone, and MDMA are fragmented in the collision cell with helium gas in the Pulsed q collision-induced dissociation (PQD) mode into m/z 134 and 117 for cathine, m/z 132 and 105 for cathinone, and m/z 163 and 135 for MDMA. The PQD values for cathine and cathinone were 19 and 22 for MDMA. Qualitative and quantitative analyses were performed using X-Caliber Software. The analytical method employed in this study was developed and validated in our laboratory, and it is already routinely used to analyze amphetamine and related substances, with in-house modifications [23].

The general unknown screening analysis was performed via gas chromatography–mass spectrometry (GC/MS) analysis (GC/MS Agilent Technologies, Santa Clara, CA, USA). Each sample (one ml of a homogenate sample) was mixed with 1 mL of the phosphate buffer (pH 6). One milliliter of the homogenate sample was extracted via the solid phase extraction (SPE) technique using DAU extraction columns (UCT, Bristol, PA, USA) according the manufacture's instructions. For instance, columns were conditioned with 3 mL of methanol and then 3 mL of deionized water and equilibrated with 1 mL of the phosphate buffer (pH 6). Two milliliters of each sample was loaded and allowed to pass slowly. Then, the columns were washed with 3 mL of deionized water followed by 1 mL of 0.1 M acetic acid and allowed to dry for 15 min under a flow of air. The first elution was collected by adding 2 mL of ethyl acetate/hexane (50:50, v:v). Thereafter, the columns were washed with 3 mL of methanol, 2 mL of the second elution (dichloromethane/isopropanol/ammonium hydroxide; 78:20:2, v:v:v) was added, and the sample was dried under nitrogen. All samples were reconstituted with methanol (100 µL), then vortexed, and transferred to GC/MS autosampler vials for GC/MS analysis.

The Thermo Fisher Scientific (TR-5MS) separation column had the following properties: 30 m length, internal diameter (ID) 0.25 mm, and film thickness 0.25 µm. Helium was used as the carrier gas with 1 mL/min flow rate. A total of 2 µL of each sample was injected into the splitless mode at an injection port with a temperature of 260 °C. The GC thermal program started at 80 °C and lasted 1.5 min. The thermal program then increased the temperature at the initial ramp to 210 °C at a rate of 30 °C/min and then slowed to 20 °C/min to reach the final temperature of 320 °C, which was held for 11 min. Electron ionization (EI) was used as the ion source in MS, and the analysis was carried out in scanning mode with an electron energy of 70 eV. The temperature of the ion source and transfer line was set at 230 °C. The mass spectral libraries from Wiley and the National Institute of Standards and Technology (NIST) were used to identify the GC/MS mass spectra of unknown substances.

2.3. Statistical Analysis

All variables were categorized and tabulated using descriptive statistics. Means, standard error of mean (SEM), and median were presented. SigmaPlot for Windows Version 11.0 was used to analyze all of the data.

3. Results

The Forensic Medicine Center in Jazan, Saudi Arabia, investigated 651 fatal cases over four-year period. Thirty of the cases had postmortem samples positive for cathinone and cathine, the active ingredients in khat. They were all males ranging in age from 23 to 45. Firearm injuries (10 cases), hanging (7 cases), road traffic accidents (2 cases), head injury (2 cases), stab wounds (2 cases), poisoning (2 cases), unknown (2 cases), ischemic heart disease (1 case), brain tumor (1 case), and choking (1 case) were responsible for the deaths. The toxicological analysis of cathinone and cathine in fatalities involving khat was performed and summarized (Tables 1 and 2).

Table 1. Postmortem toxicological analysis of cathinone in fatalities involving khat.

Specimens	Cathinone Concentrations (ng/mL)					
	Brain	Liver	Kidney	Blood	Urine	Stomach [1]
Number of samples	10	8	11	12	21	12
Mean ± SEM	69 ± 14.5	64 ± 16	43 ± 10	85 ± 26	1009 ± 204	Positive
Median	70	48	33	40	860	-
10–90 Percentile	25–126	30–138	13–99	18–218	105–2134	-

[1] The stomach results indicate exposure, not acute toxicity.

Table 2. Postmortem toxicological analysis of cathine in fatalities involving khat.

Specimens	Cathine Concentrations (ng/mL)					
	Brain	Liver	Kidney	Blood	Urine	Stomach [1]
Number of samples	13	17	16	17	22	16
Mean ± SEM	682 ± 170	635 ± 132	758 ± 167	486 ± 80	12,616 ± 3279	Positive
Median	494	430	691	470	6240	-
10–90 Percentile	227–1471	162–1140	184–1530	222–843	1790–36,400	-

[1] The stomach results indicate exposure, not acute toxicity.

The average cathinone and cathine concentrations were 85 and 486 ng/mL in the blood, 1009 and 12,616 ng/mL in the urine, 69 and 682 ng/mL in the brain, 64 and 635 ng/mL in the liver, and 43 and 758 ng/mL in the kidney. The blood concentrations of cathinone and cathine ranged from 18 to 218 ng/mL and from 222 to 843 ng/mL, respectively. In 90% of fatalities involving khat, cathinone concentrations greater than 18 ng/mL and cathine concentrations greater than 222 ng/mL were detected. The retention time for cathine, cathinone and MDMA were 4.4, 4.5, and 5.1 min, respectively. The limits of quantification (LOQ) and detection (LOD) were both 36 ng/mL. Precision and accuracy were within 20% standard deviation and 20% bias, respectively. The extraction recovery ranged from 80 to 90%, with less than 20% carryover. At doses of 100 ng/mL and 6000 ng/mL, the matrix effects (suppression/enhancement) were within the acceptable limits (25%).

The urine samples had the highest 90th percentile concentrations of cathinone (2134 ng/mL) and cathine (36,400 ng/mL). Figures 1 and 2 show box plot diagrams of the median and interquartile range of cathinone and cathine concentrations detected in fatalities involving khat. According to the current study, the number of fatalities involving khat in the last four years increased from 3% in 2018 and 2019 to 4% and 9% in 2020 and 2021, respectively.

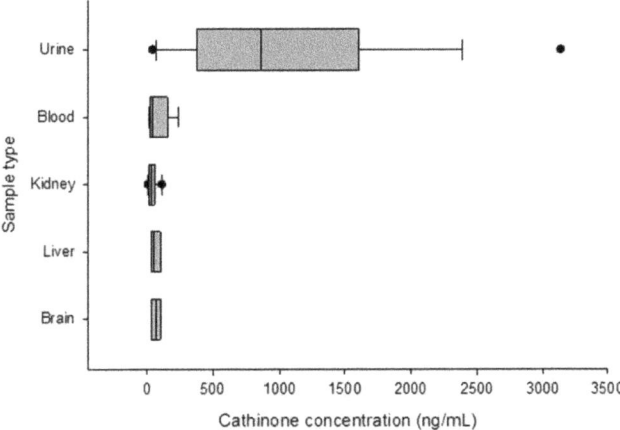

Figure 1. Box plot diagrams of the median and interquartile range of cathinone concentrations detected in fatalities involving khat. Individual dots represent outlier values.

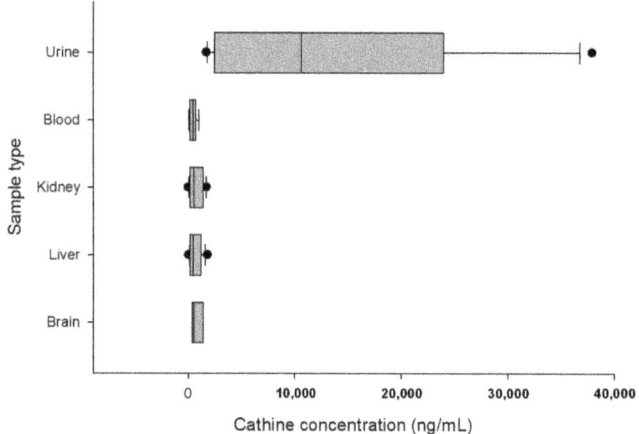

Figure 2. Box plot diagrams of the median and interquartile range of cathine concentrations detected in fatalities involving khat. Individual dots represent outlier values.

Table 3 summarizes the findings of the autopsy. Homicide was the major manner of death (13 of 30 fatalities), and firearm injuries are the leading cause of death among homicide victims (10 of 13 fatalities).

Table 3. Summary of autopsy findings.

Case Number	Age (Year)	Cause of Death	Manner of Death	Detected Drugs
1	24	Blunt trauma to head and neck (skull fractures, brain hemorrhage)	Homicidal	Cathinone, Cathine
2	24	Firearm injury in head (skull fractures and brain lacerations)	Homicidal	Cathinone, Cathine
3	24	Firearm injuries in chest (lung lacerations and hemopneumothorax) and abdomen (hepatic, intestinal, and renal lacerations)	Homicidal	Cathinone, Cathine
4	25	Stab wounds in the chest (lung lacerations and hemopneumothorax)	Homicidal	Cathinone, Cathine
5	25	Firearm injuries in head (skull fractures and brain lacerations), neck, and chest (lung lacerations)	Homicidal	Cathinone, Cathine
6	35	Firearm injuries in head (skull fractures and brain lacerations), chest (lung lacerations), and abdomen (hepatic, intestinal, and renal lacerations)	Homicidal	Cathinone, Cathine
7	26	Firearm injury in neck (major blood vessels lacerations)	Homicidal	Cathinone, Cathine
8	30	Firearm injury in chest (lung lacerations and hemopneumothorax)	Homicidal	Cathinone, Cathine
9	47	Stab wounds in the chest (lung and heart lacerations)	Homicidal	Cathinone, Cathine
10	45	Firearm injuries in chest (lung and heart lacerations) and abdomen (hepatic and renal lacerations)	Homicidal	Cathine

Table 3. Cont.

Case Number	Age (Year)	Cause of Death	Manner of Death	Detected Drugs
11	61	Firearm injuries head (skull fractures and brain lacerations) and neck	Homicidal	Cathine
12	23	Firearm injury in head (skull fractures and brain lacerations)	Homicidal	Cathine, Amphetamine
13	25	Firearm injury in head (skull fractures and brain lacerations)	Homicidal	Cathine, Amphetamine
14	23	Suicidal hanging	Suicidal	Cathinone, Cathine
15	40	Suicidal hanging	Suicidal	Cathinone, Cathine
16	23	Suicidal hanging	Suicidal	Cathinone, Cathine, Olanzapine
17	32	Suicidal hanging	Suicidal	Cathinone, Cathine, Olanzapine
18	28	Suicidal hanging	Suicidal	Cathinone, Cathine, Amphetamine
19	38	Suicidal hanging	Suicidal	Cathinone, Cathine, Amphetamine
20	25	Suicidal hanging	Suicidal	Cathinone, Cathine, Amphetamine, Ethanol, THC
21	35	Road traffic accident (skull fractures, brain injury, thoracic cage fractures)	Accidental	Cathinone, Cathine
22	29	Road traffic accident (skull fractures, brain injury, thoracic cage fractures)	Accidental	Cathinone, Cathine
23	43	Head injury (skull fracture and extradural hemorrhage)	Accidental	Cathinone, Cathine
24	25	Choking	Accidental	Cathinone, Cathine, Amphetamine
25	26	Amphetamine poisoning	Accidental	Cathinone, Cathine, Amphetamine, Dextromethorphan, Diphenhydramine
26	42	Ischemic heart disease (partial occlusion in coronaries)	Natural	Cathinone, Cathine
27	29	Brain tumor (intraventicular benign tumor)	Natural	Cathinone, Cathine, Amphetamine
28	20	Unknown	Undetermined	Cathinone, Cathine
29	28	Unknown	Undetermined	Cathinone, Cathine
30	42	Carboxy-hemoglobin poising	Undetermined	Cathine, Amphetamine

A stacked bar chart of fatalities involving khat alone or khat in combination with other drugs in different manners of death cases is presented in Figure 3. Homicide occurred more often in fatalities involving khat alone (77%) than in fatalities involving khat in combination with other drugs (23%). Suicide occurred more often in fatalities involving khat in combination with other drugs (71.5%) than in fatalities involving khat alone (28.5%).

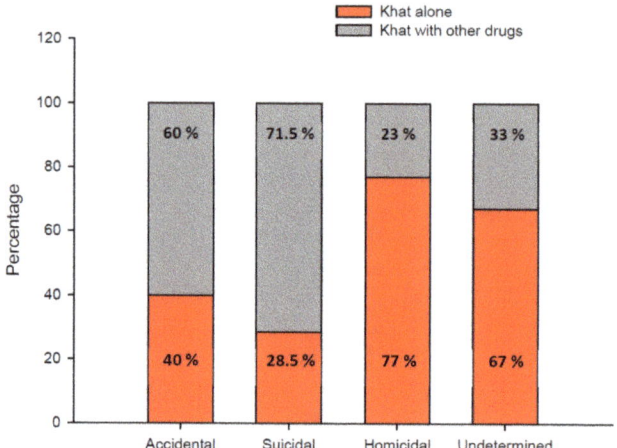

Figure 3. Stacked bar chart of occurrence of the manner of death according to fatalities involving Khat alone or Khat with other drugs.

Figure 4 is a stacked bar chart showing the occurrence of firearm injuries in fatalities involving khat (khat alone and khat with other drugs) by age group. Remarkably, all fatalities in the 20- to 30-year-old age range and more than 70 percent of fatalities in the 31- to 45-year-old age group were caused by firearm injuries in homicides involving only khat. Another remarkable finding is that five of the seven hanging suicides involved khat in combination with other drugs, and amphetamine is frequently involved in fatalities involving khat (three of seven suicide victims).

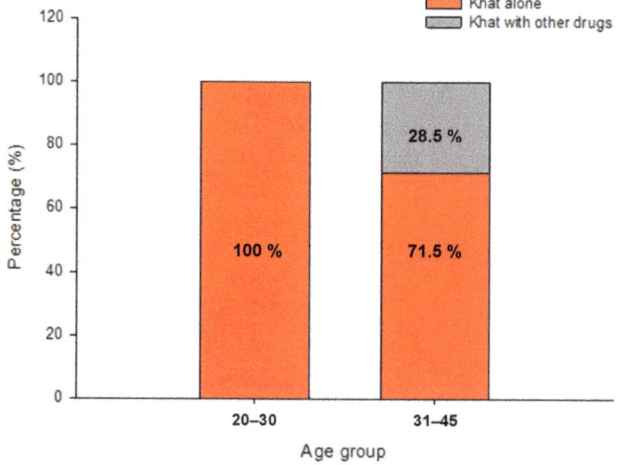

Figure 4. Stacked bar chart of occurrence of the firearm injuries in fatalities involving khat (Khat alone and Khat with other drug) by age group.

4. Discussion

The khat plant (Catha edulis (Vahl) Forssk. ex Endl.) is listed by the Saudi Food and Drugs Authority (SFDA) as a prohibited plant under the Act, whereas cathinone and cathine are listed in Schedules I and III, respectively, of the 1971 United Nations Convention on Psychotropic Substances. Khat, on the other hand, is cultivated in Yemen, where it is widely consumed. However, in the Jazan region, which is close to the Yemeni border, 21.4% of students and 28.7% of all surveyed individuals reported that they were currently chewing khat. In Yemen, khat is commonly cultivated and consumed by 68% of the surveyed Yemenis [24–26].

In 2020, khat was the most frequently seized plant-based substance, according to the United Nations Office on Drugs and Crime (UNODC, 2022). Khat accounts for 55% of all plant-based substances seized between 2016 and 2020. Saudi Arabia accounted for the most total khat seizures in 2019 [27]. In addition, chewing khat has become increasingly illegal in Europe, not because it is associated with toxicity but because it has fallen into the hands of organized crime networks [28]. There is a significant risk of toxicity for those who consume khat excessively, a problem that is common among the majority of khat users who consume large amounts of khat on a regular basis. According to a recent study, 73.5 percent of people who are dependent on khat chewing have consumed half a bundle or more of khat, and 55.9 percent of those people chew khat more than three times per week for an average of more than six hours each session [29]. Approximately 200 g of khat leaves are contained within each bundle.

Few articles have documented fatalities associated with khat, and there is currently no established reference range for cathinone and cathine that is toxic and lethal [22,30,31]. Cathinone and cathine were found in the blood, urine, vitreous humor, brain, liver, kidney, and stomach in previous studies on fatalities involving khat. Although there is no conclusive evidence that khat caused death and its presence in the body does not necessarily imply that it did, it is expected that khat will cause death when consumed in large quantities [32]. As a result, it is critical to record and publish postmortem toxicology levels in khat fatalities.

The median blood concentrations of cathinone and cathine were 40 and 470 ng/mL, respectively, exceeding the median blood levels of cathinone and cathine in previously published forensic non-fatal road traffic accidents (median 33 and 129 ng/mL, respectively; N = 19) [33]. They conclude that chewing khat may severely impair driving ability. While the median urine concentrations of cathinone and cathine were 860 and 6240 ng/mL, respectively, in our study, they were less than the median levels of cathinone and cathine in the study mentioned (median 8000 and 38,600 ng/mL, respectively; N = 19). The concentrations of drugs in the antemortem and postmortem samples are not comparable because there are more uncertainties due to variable circumstances and incomplete information, and several other factors, such as postmortem redistribution and postmortem time interval, affect tissue concentrations in autopsy samples [34–36]. This may help to explain why drug tissue concentrations in postmortem versus antemortem samples differ. Additionally, cathinone is less stable and has a shorter elimination half-life (1.5 ± 0.8 h) than cathine (5.2 ± 3.4 h) [37,38]. As a result, cathine has a longer detectable period than cathinone. Nevertheless, urine concentrations indicate chemical exposure, but not acute toxicity. On other hand, cathinone blood concentrations ranged from 19 to 122 ng/mL in forensic postmortem cases [31]. These levels were lower than the wide range observed in our study (18–218 ng/mL), while cathine blood concentration was 1447 ng/mL in one forensic postmortem case, exceeding the range observed in our study (222–843 ng/mL). The average concentrations of cathinone and cathine in the brain, liver, and kidney were 69 and 682 ng/mL, 64 and 635 ng/mL, and 43 and 758 ng/mL, respectively. The concentrations of cathine were roughly 10 times higher than those of cathinone.

Cathine and cathinone should be included in all routine toxicological investigations, especially in homicidal cases, because the number of fatalities involving khat has already increased. This study reveals the number of deaths associated with khat use, both alone and in combination with other drugs. Which demonstrate that homicidal patterns were observed in a greater proportion of cases involving khat alone (77%) than cases involving khat in combination with other drugs (23%), and that suicidal pattern was observed in a greater proportion of cases involving khat in combination with other drugs (71.5%) than cases involving khat alone (28.5%).

Khat use has been associated with a higher risk of myocardial infarction [9,39–41]. It has been shown that khat induces tachycardia and hypertension, which may be increased at a higher dose, hence raising the risk of myocardial infarction [37,42,43]. Cathine and cathinone were the only substances detected in Case 26 of the current study, which showed ischemic heart disease with coronary partial occlusion.

Hepatotoxicity, on the other hand, has been observed in multiple studies, particularly among chronic khat chewers. Multilobular necrosis, canalicular cholestasis, an enlarged liver with decreased echogenicity, cirrhotic and portal fibrosis, jaundice with elevated liver enzymes, and severe liver injury with an elevated international normalized ratio were all characteristics of khat-related hepatic toxicity [44–46]. Hepatotoxicity was cured in two cases by discontinuing khat usage [10]. In the current study, cathine and cathinone were detected in the liver at average concentrations of 635 ± 132 and 64 ± 16 ng/mL, respectively. However, no evidence of liver toxicity was found.

Khat use has also been associated with mental disorders including anxiety, irritability, aggression, psychosis, paranoia, dysphoria, depression, insomnia, hallucinations, and delusions [47–49]. In addition, anxiety, trembling, lethargy, depression, and nightmares could be withdrawal symptoms [22,50,51]. On the other hand, khat intake may aggravate schizophrenia symptoms and diminish the therapeutic efficacy of antipsychotic drugs [52]. With both khat use and withdrawal condition, incidents of violence have been reported. In addition, anxiousness and poor decision-making have been observed following khat use [29,53,54]. Repeated oral administration of khat extract, according to Banjaw et al. (2006)'s report, makes experimental rats more aggressive [55]. Moreover, studies show that khat affects driving, social behavior, and work performance. It has been associated with homicide, notably in mentally ill people [11,48,53,56,57], and two reported homicides have been linked to khat consumption [56,58].

In the current study, homicide and suicide were the leading manners of death in fatalities involving khat alone and khat in combination with other drugs, respectively. In fatalities involving khat in combination with other drugs, particularly amphetamine, suicide was the most common manner of death. This study has limitations due to the small sample size and the fact that only non-natural cases were sent for toxicological analysis. In addition, it is essential to determine the relationship between khat consumption, violent crime, and fatalities. Therefore, a study is now underway to examine the role of khat in the toxicology of violent death over a ten-year period (2014 to 2023) and to establish reference ranges for cathinone and cathine in fatalities involving khat, which will represent only the fatal cases intoxicated with both cathinone and cathine.

In spite of the limitations described above, these findings suggest that fatalities involving khat are cause for concern, particularly among young people with a higher propensity for homicide and firearm injuries. Therefore, any health-based crime prevention strategy in Jazan has to consider khat use.

5. Conclusions

This study determined the average levels of cathinone and cathine in 30 cases of fatalities involving khat. This information may help forensic toxicologists and pathologists interpret toxicological investigations, but it should not be interpreted independently of other evidence, such as the death investigation and autopsy results. To create the body of literature necessary for more precise determinations of the role of khat in crimes and death investigations, additional research is required, particularly involving toxicological investigative and autopsy findings.

Author Contributions: Conceptualization, G.S., I.A., M.G. (Mohammed Gaballah) and A.A.; methodology, M.O., S.A., M.G., I.A. and M.G.; software, I.A. and M.O.; validation, M.O., M.G. and S.A.; formal analysis, M.O. and I.A.; investigation, G.S., A.A., M.O., S.A., M.G., A.H., M.G. (Mohammed Ghalibi), M.T., M.A. and M.F.; resources, I.K., M.T. and I.A.; data curation, G.S., A.A., M.G. and I.A.; writing—original draft preparation, I.A.; writing—review and editing, G.S., M.A., M.G. and I.A.; visualization, M.G. and I.A.; supervision, I.A. and G.S.; project administration, I.A. All authors have read and agreed to the published version of the manuscript.

Funding: This research received no external funding.

Institutional Review Board Statement: This study has been reviewed and approved by Jazan Health Ethics Committee, Saudi Arabia (No. 2238).

Informed Consent Statement: Not applicable.

Data Availability Statement: All relevant details are included in the article.

Acknowledgments: The Ministry of Health's Forensic Medical Center in Jazan, Saudi Arabia, contributed substantially to this work.

Conflicts of Interest: The authors declare no conflict of interest.

References

1. Nencini, P.; Ahmed, A.M. Khat consumption: A pharmacological review. *Drug Alcohol Depend.* **1989**, *23*, 19–29. [CrossRef]
2. Drug Enforcement Administration. *Drugs of Abuse: A Dea Resource Guide*; CreateSpace Independent Publishing Platform: Scotts Valley, CA, USA, 2020.
3. Dewick, P.M. *Medicinal Natural Products: A Biosynthetic Approach*; Wiley: Hoboken, NJ, USA, 2009.
4. Halbach, H. Medical aspects of the chewing of khat leaves. *Bull. World Health Organ.* **1972**, *47*, 21.
5. Al-Habori, M. The potential adverse effects of habitual use of *Catha edulis* (khat). *Expert Opin. Drug Saf.* **2005**, *4*, 1145–1154. [CrossRef] [PubMed]
6. Kalix, P. Khat: Scientific knowledge and policy issues. *Br. J. Addict.* **1987**, *82*, 47–53. [CrossRef] [PubMed]
7. Silva, B.; Soares, J.; Rocha-Pereira, C.; Mladěnka, P.; Remião, F.; Researchers, O.B.O.T.O. Khat, a Cultural Chewing Drug: A Toxicokinetic and Toxicodynamic Summary. *Toxins* **2022**, *14*, 71. [CrossRef]
8. Saha, S.; Dollery, C. Severe Ischaemic Cardiomyopathy Associated with Khat Chewing. *J. R. Soc. Med.* **2006**, *99*, 316–318. [CrossRef]
9. Al-Motarreb, A.; Briancon, S.; Al-Jaber, N.; Al-Adhi, B.; Al-Jailani, F.; Salek, M.S.; Broadley, K. Khat chewing is a risk factor for acute myocardial infarction: A case-control study. *Br. J. Clin. Pharmacol.* **2005**, *59*, 574–581. [CrossRef] [PubMed]
10. Jenkins, M.G.; Handslip, R.; Kumar, M.; Mahadeva, U.; Lucas, S.; Yamamoto, T.; Wood, D.M.; Wong, T.; Dargan, P.I. Reversible khat-induced hepatitis: Two case reports and review of the literature. *Front. Gastroenterol.* **2013**, *4*, 278–281. [CrossRef]
11. Cox, G.; Rampes, H. Adverse effects of khat: A review. *Adv. Psychiatr. Treat.* **2003**, *9*, 456–463. [CrossRef]
12. Geisshüsler, S.; Brenneisen, R. The content of psychoactive phenylpropyl and phenylpentenyl khatamines in Catha edulis Forsk. of different origin. *J. Ethnopharmacol.* **1987**, *19*, 269–277. [CrossRef]
13. Kalix, P. Khat: A plant with amphetamine effects. *J. Subst. Abus. Treat.* **1988**, *5*, 163–169. [CrossRef]
14. Kalix, P. Cathinone, a natural amphetamine. *Pharmacol. Toxicol.* **1992**, *70*, 77–86. [CrossRef]
15. Nencini, P.; Ahmed, A.M.; Amiconi, G.; Elmi, A.S. Tolerance Develops to Sympathetic Effects of Khat in Humans. *Pharmacology* **1984**, *28*, 150–154. [CrossRef]
16. Bedada, W.; de Andrés, F.; Engidawork, E.; Pohanka, A.; Beck, O.; Bertilsson, L.; Llerena, A.; Aklillu, E. The Psychostimulant Khat (Catha edulis) Inhibits CYP2D6 Enzyme Activity in Humans. *J. Clin. Psychopharmacol.* **2015**, *35*, 694–699. [CrossRef] [PubMed]
17. Bedada, W.; de Andrés, F.; Engidawork, E.; Hussein, J.; Llerena, A.; Aklillu, E. Effects of Khat (Catha edulis) use on catalytic activities of major drug-metabolizing cytochrome P450 enzymes and implication of pharmacogenetic variations. *Sci. Rep.* **2018**, *8*, 12726. [CrossRef] [PubMed]
18. Pélissier-Alicot, A.-L.; Gaulier, J.-M.; Champsaur, P.; Marquet, P. Mechanisms Underlying Postmortem Redistribution of Drugs: A Review. *J. Anal. Toxicol.* **2003**, *27*, 533–544. [CrossRef]
19. Tseng, Y.L.; Shieh, M.-H.; Kuo, F.-H. Metabolites of ephedrines in human urine after administration of a single therapeutic dose. *Forensic Sci. Int.* **2006**, *157*, 149–155. [CrossRef]
20. Pokrajac, M.; Miljković, B.; Bisailović, B. Mass spectrometric investigation of 2-aminopropiophenones and some of their metabolites. *Rapid Commun. Mass Spectrom.* **1991**, *5*, 59–61. [CrossRef]
21. Scheline, R.R. *Handbook of Mammalian Metabolism of Plant Compounds*; CRC Press: Boca Raton, FL, USA, 2017.
22. Oyefeso, A.; Naidoo, V.; Schifano, F.; Tonia, T.; Corkery, J.M.; Button, J.; Ghodse, A.H. Overview of literature and information on "khat-related" mortality: A call for recognition of the issue and further research. *Ann. Dell'istituto Super. Di Sanità* **2011**, *47*, 445–464. [CrossRef]

23. Alamir, A.; Watterson, J.; Attafi, I. Development and Validation of a Uplc-Qtof-Ms Method for Blood Analysis of Isomeric Amphetamine-Related Drugs. *Separations* **2022**, *9*, 285. [CrossRef]
24. Alsanosy, R.; Mahfouz, M.S.; Gaffar, A. Khat Chewing Habit among School Students of Jazan Region, Saudi Arabia. *PLoS ONE* **2013**, *8*, e65504. [CrossRef]
25. Ageely, H.M. Prevalence of Khat chewing in college and secondary (high) school students of Jazan region, Saudi Arabia. *Harm Reduct. J.* **2009**, *6*, 11–17. [CrossRef]
26. Numan, N. Exploration of adverse psychological symptoms in Yemeni khat users by the Symptoms Checklist-90 (SCL-90). *Addiction* **2003**, *99*, 61–65. [CrossRef]
27. The United Nations Office on Drugs and Crime (UNODC). *Drug Market Trends of Cocaine, Amphetamine-Type Stimulants and New Psychoactive Substances*; United Nations Publication: Vienna, Austria, 2022; ISBN 9789211483758.
28. Karch, S.B.; Drummer, O. *Karch's Pathology of Drug Abuse*; Taylor & Francis: Abingdon, UK, 2015.
29. El-Setouhy, M.; Alsanosy, R.M.; Alsharqi, A.; Ismail, A.A. Khat Dependency and Psychophysical Symptoms among Chewers in Jazan Region, Kingdom of Saudi Arabia. *BioMed Res. Int.* **2016**, *2016*, 2642506. [CrossRef]
30. Attafi, I.M.; Albeishy, M.Y.; Oraiby, M.E.; Khardali, I.A.; Shaikhain, G.A.; Fageeh, M.M. Postmortem Distribution of Cathinone and Cathine in Human Biological Specimens in a Case of Death Associated with Khat Chewing. *Arab. J. Forensic Sci. Forensic Med.* **2018**, *1*, 922–930. [CrossRef]
31. Corkery, J.M.; Schifano, F.; Oyefeso, A.; Ghodse, A.H.; Tonia, T.; Naidoo, V.; Button, J. 'Bundle of fun' or 'bunch of problems'? Case series of khat-related deaths in the UK. *Drugs Educ. Prev. Policy* **2011**, *18*, 408–425. [CrossRef]
32. Corkery, J.M. Khat—Chewing It Over: Continuing 'Cultural Cement', Cardiac Challenge or Catalyst for Change. In *Forensic Toxicology–Drug Use and Misuse*; Royal Society of Chemistry: London, UK, 2016; pp. 165–207.
33. Toennes, S.W.; Kauert, G.F. Driving under the influence of khat—Alkaloid concentrations and observations in forensic cases. *Forensic Sci. Int.* **2004**, *140*, 85–90. [CrossRef] [PubMed]
34. Patel, G. Postmortem Drug Levels: Innocent Bystander or Guilty as Charged. *J. Pharm. Pract.* **2012**, *25*, 37–40. [CrossRef]
35. Prouty, R.; Anderson, W.H. The forensic science implications of site and temporal influences on postmortem blood-drug concentrations. *J. Forensic Sci.* **1990**, *35*, 243–270. [CrossRef]
36. Yarema, M.C.; Becker, C.E. Key Concepts in Postmortem Drug Redistribution. *Clin. Toxicol.* **2005**, *43*, 235–241. [CrossRef]
37. Toennes, S.W.; Harder, S.; Schramm, M.; Niess, C.; Kauert, G.F. Pharmacokinetics of cathinone, cathine and norephedrine after the chewing of khat leaves. *Br. J. Clin. Pharmacol.* **2003**, *56*, 125–130. [CrossRef] [PubMed]
38. Widler, P.; Mathys, K.; Brenneisen, R.; Kalix, P.; Fisch, H.-U. Pharmacodynamics and pharmacokinetics of khat: A controlled study. *Clin. Pharmacol. Ther.* **1994**, *55*, 556–562. [CrossRef] [PubMed]
39. Al-Motarreb, A.; Shabana, A.; El-Menyar, A. Epicardical Coronary Arteries in Khat Chewers Presenting with Myocardial Infarction. *Int. J. Vasc. Med.* **2013**, *2013*, 857019. [CrossRef] [PubMed]
40. Alkadi, H.O.; Noman, M.A.; Al-Thobhani, A.K.; Al-Mekhlafi, F.S.; Raja'a, Y.A. Clinical and experimental evaluation of the effect of Khat-induced myocardial infarction. *Saudi Med. J.* **2002**, *23*, 1195–1198.
41. Al-Hashem, F.H.; Dallak, M.A.; Nwoye, L.O.; Bin-Jaliah, I.M.; Al-Amri, H.S.; Rezk, M.H.; Sakr, H.F.; Shatoor, A.S.; Al-Khateeb, M. Acute exposure to Catha edulis depresses contractility and induces myocardial infarction in spontaneously contracting, isolated rabbit's heart. *Saudi J. Biol. Sci.* **2012**, *19*, 93–101. [CrossRef]
42. Al-Motarreb, A.L.; Broadley, K. Coronary and aortic vasoconstriction by cathinone, the active constituent of khat. *Auton. Autacoid Pharmacol.* **2003**, *23*, 319–326. [CrossRef]
43. Al-Motarreb, A.; Al-Kebsi, M.; Al-Adhi, B.; Broadley, K.J. Khat chewing and acute myocardial infarction. *Heart* **2002**, *87*, 279–280. [CrossRef]
44. Peevers, C.G.; Moorghen, M.; Collins, P.L.; Gordon, F.H.; McCune, C.A. Liver disease and cirrhosis because of Khat chewing in UK Somali men: A case series. *Liver Int.* **2010**, *30*, 1242–1243. [CrossRef]
45. Chapman, M.H.; Kajihara, M.; Borges, G.; O'Beirne, J.; Patch, D.; Dhillon, A.P.; Crozier, A.; Morgan, M.Y. Severe, Acute Liver Injury and Khat Leaves. *N. Engl. J. Med.* **2010**, *362*, 1642–1644. [CrossRef]
46. Brostoff, J.; Plymen, C.; Birns, J. Khat—A novel cause of drug-induced hepatitis. *Eur. J. Intern. Med.* **2006**, *17*, 383. [CrossRef]
47. Balint, E.E.; Falkay, G.; Balint, G.A. Khat–a controversial plant. *Wien. Klin. Wochenschr.* **2009**, *121*, 604–614. [CrossRef]
48. Pantelis, C.; Hindler, C.G.; Taylor, J.C. Use and abuse of khat (*Catha edulis*): A review of the distribution, pharmacology, side effects and a description of psychosis attributed to khat chewing. *Psychol. Med.* **1989**, *19*, 657–668. [CrossRef]
49. Odenwald, M. Chronic khat use and psychotic disorders: A review of the literature and future prospects. *Sucht* **2007**, *53*, 9–22. [CrossRef]
50. Wabel, N.T. Psychopharmacological aspects of catha edulis (khat) and consequences of long term use: A review. *Psychiatry Behav. Sci.* **2011**, *1*, 187. [CrossRef]
51. Giannini, A.J.; Castellani, S. A Manic-like Psychosis Due to Khat Catha edulis Forsk. *J. Toxicol. Clin. Toxicol.* **1982**, *19*, 455–459. [CrossRef]
52. Hakami, T.; Mahmoud, M.; Mohammed, B.; El-Setouhy, M. Effects of khat use on response to antipsychotic medications in patients with newly diagnosed schizophrenia: A retrospective study. *East. Mediterr. Health J.* **2021**, *27*, 353–360. [CrossRef] [PubMed]

53. Odenwald, M.; Neuner, F.; Schauer, M.; Elbert, T.; Catani, C.; Lingenfelder, B.; Hinkel, H.; Häfner, H.; Rockstroh, B. Khat use as risk factor for psychotic disorders: A cross-sectional and case-control study in Somalia. *BMC Med.* **2005**, *3*, 5. [CrossRef]
54. Gelaye, B.; Philpart, M.; Goshu, M.; Berhane, Y.; Fitzpatrick, A.L.; Williams, M.A. Anger expression, negative life events and violent behaviour among male college students in Ethiopia. *Scand. J. Public Health* **2008**, *36*, 538–545. [CrossRef] [PubMed]
55. Banjaw, M.Y.; Miczek, K.; Schmidt, W.J. Repeated Catha edulis oral administration enhances the baseline aggressive behavior in isolated rats. *J. Neural Transm.* **2005**, *113*, 543–556. [CrossRef] [PubMed]
56. Alem, A.; Shibre, T. Khat induced psychosis and its medico-legal implication: A case report. *Ethiop. Med J.* **1997**, *35*, 137–139. [PubMed]
57. Khat Chewing: An Emerging Drug Concern in Australia? *Aust. N. Z. J. Psychiatry* **2005**, *39*, 842–843. [CrossRef] [PubMed]
58. Tesfaye, E.; Krahl, W.; Alemayehu, S. Khat induced psychotic disorder: Case report. *Subst. Abus. Treat. Prev. Policy* **2020**, *15*, 27. [CrossRef] [PubMed]

Disclaimer/Publisher's Note: The statements, opinions and data contained in all publications are solely those of the individual author(s) and contributor(s) and not of MDPI and/or the editor(s). MDPI and/or the editor(s) disclaim responsibility for any injury to people or property resulting from any ideas, methods, instructions or products referred to in the content.

MDPI
St. Alban-Anlage 66
4052 Basel
Switzerland
www.mdpi.com

Toxics Editorial Office
E-mail: toxics@mdpi.com
www.mdpi.com/journal/toxics

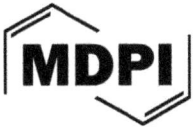

Disclaimer/Publisher's Note: The statements, opinions and data contained in all publications are solely those of the individual author(s) and contributor(s) and not of MDPI and/or the editor(s). MDPI and/or the editor(s) disclaim responsibility for any injury to people or property resulting from any ideas, methods, instructions or products referred to in the content.

www.ingramcontent.com/pod-product-compliance
Lightning Source LLC
LaVergne TN
LVHW070558100526
838202LV00012B/501